Documentation for

PHYSICIAN ASSISTANTS

Documentation for
PHYSICIAN ASSISTANTS

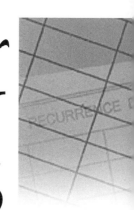

Debra D. Sullivan, PhD, PA-C
Program Director and Associate Professor
Physician Assistant Program
Midwestern University
Glendale, Arizona

and

Lynnette J. Mattingly, MHPE, PA-C
Adjunct Clinical Faculty
Physician Assistant Program
Midwestern University
Glendale, Arizona

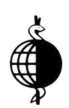

F.A. DAVIS COMPANY • Philadelphia

F. A. Davis Company
1915 Arch Street
Philadelphia, PA 19103
www.fadavis.com

Printed in the United States of America

Last digit indicates print number: 10 9 8 7 6 5 4 3

Publisher: Margaret M. Biblis
Acquisitions Editor: Carl Holm
Manager, Creative Development: Susan Rhyner
Developmental Editor: Peg Waltner

As new scientific information becomes available through basic and clinical research, recommended treatments and drug therapies undergo changes. The author(s) and publisher have done everything possible to make this book accurate, up to date, and in accord with accepted standards at the time of publication. The author(s), editors, and publisher are not responsible for errors or omissions or for consequences from application of the book, and make no warranty, expressed or implied, in regard to the contents of the book. Any practice described in this book should be applied by the reader in accordance with professional standards of care used in regard to the unique circumstances that may apply in each situation. The reader is advised always to check product information (package inserts) for changes and new information regarding dose and contraindications before administering any drug. Caution is especially urged when using new or infrequently ordered drugs.

Dedication

We dedicate this book to the mentors who have taught
us over the years, to the students who teach us every day, and to all
Physician Assistants, present and future, who strive to deliver quality care.

Introduction

You might be asking, "Why a book on documentation?" Documentation is one of the most important skills a Physician Assistant (PA) or any other healthcare provider can learn. You might feel tempted to focus considerably more time and energy on learning other skills, such as physical examination, suturing, pharmacotherapeutics, etc. These are essential skills, but we also want to stress to you that documentation likewise is extremely important. State licensure laws and regulations, accrediting bodies, professional association guidelines, and federal reimbursement programs all require that healthcare providers maintain a record for each of their patients.

Your documentation establishes your credibility as a healthcare provider. Other providers will assess your ability to adequately reflect a patient's care through the medical record. Other healthcare providers will assume, rightly or wrongly, that you practice medicine much in the same manner as that in which you document. If your documentation is sloppy, full of errors, or incomplete, others will assume that is the way you practice. Alternately, thorough, legible, and complete documentation will give others that impression of your credibility. Some excellent providers simply do not have good documentation skills. However, this is the exception, not the rule. It is very difficult to persuade those who read sloppy documentation that the person who wrote that way can and did provide good care.

All medical records are legal documents and are important for both the healthcare provider and the patient, regardless of where the patient care takes place. The most important legal functions of medical records are to provide evidence that appropriate care was given and to document the patient's response to that care. There is a well-established principle of documentation that every healthcare provider should remember: if it is not documented, it was not done. This might seem harsh in some respects, but consider the tremendous time lapse between when events occur (and when they are documented) and when litigation occurs. It might be anywhere from 2 to 7 years from occurrence of an event until you are called to give a sworn account of the event. The medical record is usually the only detailed record of what actually occurred, and only what is written is considered to have occurred. You will not remember the details of an event that happened 6 years ago, and your only memory aid will be the medical record. As a legal document, plaintiff attorneys, defense attorneys, malpractice carriers, jurors, judges, and most likely the patient might have access to medical records you author. You should keep this in mind at all times when documenting.

Many reviewers from various organizations can obtain access to the medical record for a variety of purposes. Representatives from insurance companies or state or federal payers can review the record for purposes of deciding on payment or looking for evidence of fraud and abuse. Peer review organizations might review the record to determine if the care reflected in your documentation is consistent with the standard of care. Researchers often obtain access to medical records for purposes of conducting scientific research.

Throughout this book, you will analyze examples of documentation. You may also complete the worksheets, which will help you apply the information you have just read. The purpose of this book is to teach documentation skills, not the practice of medicine. The content of a medical record varies greatly, depending on the patient's presenting problem or condition; however, the process of documenting the information does not vary greatly, so our focus is on the process.

We assume that you already have some knowledge of commonly used medical abbreviations, but we have used abbreviations throughout the book and have incorporated them into the chapter worksheets. We offer one caution about using abbreviations: always be clear about your intended meaning. For example, if you use the abbreviation "CP," one person could read that as "chest pain" and another as "cerebral palsy". Of course, the rest of the entry should make it clear which term the abbreviation is being used for.

Acknowledgments

We thank our colleagues at Midwestern University for their unwavering support and friendship during the writing of this book. For her assistance, the authors especially thank our contributor: Kristin Foulke, MPH, PA-C, Instructor, Physician Assistant Program, Midwestern University, Glendale, Arizona. We are also indebted to those students who offered suggestions and a fresh perspective on our work. Most important, we acknowledge the love and support of our husbands, Greg Sullivan and Bill Mattingly, and their encouragement on this journey that we have taken together.

We thank Sue Pringle, F.A. Davis representative, who saw a spark, and Margaret Biblis, Acquisitions Editor, who fanned the spark into a flame. We are indebted to Carl Holm, acquisitions editor, and Susan Rhyner, development editor, both with F.A. Davis, for answering our many questions and guiding us through the problems of first-time authors. Peg Waltner, developmental editor, was an absolute lifesaver who came to our aid again and again; without her guidance, this project would never have been completed. We also extend our gratitude to Scott Filderman, Project Editor at F.A. Davis, for his work with the manuscript, and to Samuel Rondinelli, Production Manager. We extend special thanks to Dr. Suzanne M. Bennett, our supervising physician, colleague, and friend, who shared with us her expertise and forms.

Debbie Sullivan and Lynnette Mattingly

Reviewers

The authors would like to thank the following educators for their careful review:

Steven Bents, MPAS, PA-C
Program Director
Rocky Mountain College
Billings, MT

Winston Hunt, PA-C
Assistant Professor
Medical College of Georgia
Augusta, GA

Pat Kenney-Moore, MS, PA-C
Associate Director – Academic Coordinator
Oregon Health Sciences University
Portland, OR

Cynthia Lord, PA-C
Professor
Quinnipiac University
Cheshire, CT

Dawn B. Ludwig, PHD, PA-C
Associate Professor – Program Director
Augsburg College
Minneapolis, MN

Ann Mekilo, MS, PA-C
Clinical Director
Marywood University
Scranton, PA

Contents

SOAP Notes

■ Purpose

Section 1 teaches you how to document subjective and objective information, assessment of a patient's problem, and the plan of care for that patient using the SOAP note format. This format is widely used to document patient encounters in various settings and presents information systematically and logically. A complete history is usually obtained when a person presents as a new patient to a practice setting; it should be reviewed and updated at least annually. The SOAP note itself is rarely used to record a patient's entire medical history. It is widely used in ambulatory care settings for episodic or problem-specific visits and in inpatient settings to document the patient's daily progress or condition. One chapter is devoted to each component of the SOAP format.

■ Objectives

- Provide 10 helpful basic principles for charting and documentation.
- Define the subjective, objective, assessment, and plan components.
- Organize data using the SOAP format.
- Organize pertinent positive and negative aspects of the history and physical examination.
- Document assessments using terminology consistent with ICD-10 codes.

- Understand how documentation of ICD-10 codes supports the level of care provided.
- Document components of the management plan.
- Use information to complete worksheets.

It is necessary here to discuss 10 basic principles of charting and documentation. These are principles, not hard and fast rules. Some institutions have their own regulations about documentation, so it is a good idea to find out what regulations are in place at your institution. If none have been established, this summary is a good place to start.

1. When writing, always use permanent ink. Black ink is usually preferred, because it reproduces best on copies.

2. All entries in a record should be noted by date and time. In most hospital settings, military time is preferred (i.e., 2 p.m. is 1400).

3. Each entry should conclude with your signature and, when necessary, should be signed by a preceptor/supervising physician.

4. Each entry should be legible.

5. Never alter an entry for any reason. Never use correction fluid or cover over an entry in any manner. The original entry should be entirely readable. If a mistake is made, draw a single line through the error, label as an error, and if space allows, make the correction in the same area of the note. If there is not sufficient space

to make the correction, it should be entered as an addendum to the original note. The error and the correction, and the addendum if necessary, should be initialed, and time and date of the correction should be noted. Avoid trying to squeeze in words, resulting in an illegible entry.

6. If something is omitted from an entry, do not add the information to the original note. Make a separate entry labeled "late entry," then include date and time as usual.

7. Do not leave blank lines between entries.

8. Use only standard medical abbreviations.

9. Maintain confidentiality of records at all times. Be careful not to leave the record in an area where others who should not have access to the record may read it.

10. Never release any information from the medical record to anyone unless proper "consent to release information" has been given by the patient (or parent or legal guardian if patient is a minor or is incapacitated). Each office or hospital should have its own policy and procedure for release of medical records, and it is your responsibility to know and follow these.

Chapter 1

Subjective

$\mathcal{T}$he subjective portion of the SOAP (Subjective, Objective, Assessment, Plan) note is information that the subject tells you. Think of it as the patient's story: it will comprise all the history the patient tells you. Sometimes, subjective (S) information is obtained from someone other than the patient. A spouse or family member, a caregiver, nursing staff or other healthcare providers could all offer subjective information. The patient's prior medical record is another potential source. The completeness and accuracy of the history (the subjective information) will help guide what you look for when performing a problem-specific physical examination (the objective information) and formulating differential diagnoses. Together, the subjective and objective (O) information should lead you to and should support the assessment (A). Once you have made an assessment, you can establish a plan (P) of care.

It is beyond the scope of this book to address interviewing techniques and interpersonal skills; you should employ your best communication techniques when interviewing the patient and obtaining the history that will make up the subjective portion of the SOAP note. Keep in mind that you will make an assessment (or diagnosis) based on history alone in about 75% of patient encounters; therefore, gathering and documenting the information appropriately is critical. On occasion, you might want to use quotation marks to identify information as a direct quote from the patient and that you have recorded their exact words. This technique is particularly useful if the patient describes something important (such as pain) or if the patient does not answer a question to your satisfaction. For instance, when asked if she takes any medication, a patient responds "Yes, I take a little red pill for my blood pressure." You could guess what that little red pill may be, but for the sake of accuracy, it would probably be better to document using the patient's words (patient takes "a little red pill" for hypertension). The use of quotation marks lets other readers know the information within the marks is not your paraphrase or restatement of something the patient told you but the words of the patient.

Scope of Subjective Information

Subjective information includes the following information:

- Chief complaint (CC)
- History of present illness (HPI)
- Pertinent past medical history (PMH)
- Pertinent family history (FH)
- Pertinent social history (SH)
- Pertinent psychiatric history
- Cultural history
- Any specialized history related to the chief complaint (for instance, obstetrical and gynecological history for a female patient who presents with irregular menses)
- Pertinent review of systems (ROS)

Table 1–1 gives the details of each section of the complete history. See also Figures 5–1 and 5–2.

Although content is more important than form, the subjective information is usually documented in the order listed above. Note that physical examination findings are not

Table 1–1 Components of a Complete History

Section of the History	Information Included
Chief complaint	The main reason why the patient is seeking care
History of present illness	The seven cardinal attributes:
	1. Onset and duration
	2. Location
	3. Character
	4. Severity
	5. Associated signs and symptoms
	6. Aggravating factors
	7. Alleviating factors
Past medical history	Current and/or chronic medical conditions
	Previous surgeries and whether or not patient has received any blood transfusions
	Current medications
	Allergies
	Immunization status
	Health maintenance status
	Preventive care
	For females, obstetrical and gynecological history
Family history	Age and current health condition of living parents, siblings, and children.
	For family members that are deceased, age at death and cause.
	Presence of diseases with a familial tendency.
Social history	Marital status, occupation or student status, living arrangements, education, sexual orientation, habits such as tobacco, alcohol or drug use.
Psychiatric history	Current mental state, history of depression or other mental disorders, history of suicide threat or attempt.
Cultural history	Patient's belief system as to cause of illness; family dynamics and authority within family; spiritual/religious practices; taboos.
Any specialized history related to the chief complain	Obstetrical and gynecological history for a female patient, prenatal history for an infant, course of a chronic disease, etc.
Review of systems [Head, Eyes, Ears, Nose, and Throat (HEENT)]	General: weight gain or loss, activity level, fever, chills, sweats.
	HEENT: change in hearing, vision, smell, taste; pain or discomfort in ears, eyes, nose, throat, sinuses; persistent or uncharacteristic headaches; nasal discharge, change in voice.
	Neck: swollen glands or other areas of swelling, restriction of movement.
	Respiratory: shortness of breath, cough, dyspnea on exertion, hemoptysis, orthopnea.
	Cardiovascular: chest pain with or without exertion, chest wall pain, venous distention, swelling of feet and/or hands
	[Gastrointestinal (GI)] GI: change in appetite, difficulty chewing or swallowing, nausea, vomiting, diarrhea, constipation, cramping, bloating, indigestion, blood in stool, hemorrhoids.
	[Genitourinary (GU)] GU: pain with urination, hesitancy, frequency, hematuria
	Reproductive: irregular menses, painful menses, vaginal pain or discharge, dyspareunia, penile discharge, testicular or scrotal pain or swelling
	Musculoskeletal: range of motion of joints, joint pain or swelling, redness or warmth of a joint
	Hematological: easy bruising, bleeding from gums, delayed wound healing, recurrent infections
	Psychiatric: affective or personality disorders, depressed mood, sleep disturbances, suicidal ideation, hallucination, illusions, delusions, substance abuse.

documented in the subjective section; these findings are objective information.

One of the most challenging aspects of documenting the subjective information is determining what elements of the history are pertinent. It takes years of practicing medicine to understand the importance of certain associated signs and symptoms and how they relate to the chief complaint and to understand how the onset, location, character, and severity of pain represent a certain condition. Some data from the history will support or suggest one diagnosis more than another. These data are "pertinent positives." The absence of other data, called "pertinent negatives," likewise will suggest a certain diagnosis and help rule out other diagnoses. When documenting certain areas of the history, such as associated signs and symptoms, it is helpful to list all pertinent positives together, and then list the pertinent negatives. For example, a patient presents with the chief complaint of a sore throat. A pertinent positive is that the patient has a fever. A pertinent negative is that the patient has not had stiffness of the neck or drooling. The documentation of pertinent positives and negatives should be detailed enough to narrow the differential diagnoses and eventually lead to the most likely diagnosis. Try to anticipate what information other readers want to know, and be sure that information is included in your documentation.

Application Exercise 1.1

Read the following paragraph and answer the questions that follow.
A 45-year-old-woman presents with a chief complaint of right hand pain. List the 7 cardinal aspects of the history of present illness that should be documented in the subjective information.

_____

_____

_____

_____

_____

_____

List several pertinent aspects of the PMH that should be documented.

_____

_____

_____

What information about the patient's social history would be important to document?

_____

_____

_____

APPLICATION EXERCISE 1.1 ANSWERS

1. Onset and duration
2. Location
3. Character
4. Severity
5. Associated signs and symptoms
6. Aggravating factors
7. Alleviating factors

List several pertinent aspects of the PMH that should be documented:
Medical history, surgical history, allergies, current medications
What information about the patient's social history would be important to document?
Occupational history (to determine if hand pain is related to job activities)
Tobacco use, alcohol use, and recreational drug use are usually documented for every patient.

Development of Documentation Skills

There are at least two ways to develop documentation skills: (1) practice, practice, and practice and (2) critically analyze documentation. We give you the opportunity to do both throughout this text. Read the subjective information documented in the following two examples, and answer the questions.

EXAMPLE 1–1

This 42-year-old man presents with left knee pain. He injured his knee while playing softball. His pain has gradually worsened over the past week. He has not

(Continued)

EXAMPLE 1–1 *(Continued)*

noticed any swelling. He denies any numbness below the knee. No prior knee surgery. Allergic to penicillin. Denies tobacco use. Works full-time in computer sales.

After reading this example, try to answer the following questions:

1. How long has the patient had left knee pain?

2. Has he tried anything to relieve the pain?

3. What pertinent positives and negatives are documented? Should any other pertinent elements have been documented?

4. Does the patient have any chronic medical conditions?

5. Has the patient had any surgery?

6. Does the patient take any medications?

As you can see, this entry did not allow you to answer these questions. However, the information should be part of the history related to the patient's chief complaint of knee pain and should be documented as subjective information. This information is important to anyone who may be involved in the patient's care. Read Example 1–2, and then answer these same questions.

EXAMPLE 1–2

This 42-year-old man presents with complaints of left knee pain. He originally injured his left knee about a month ago while playing softball. In the past week, the pain has gradually worsened. He describes the pain as "a deep ache." He has not noted any swelling of the knee. The pain is worse when he has to stand for more than a half hour at a time and when he walks and goes upstairs. The patient has taken ibuprofen 400 mg occasionally for the pain, with some relief. He denies any numbness or tingling of the extremity or previous injury to the knee. He does not have any chronic medical problems and specifically denies having a history of hypertension or ulcers. He has never had surgery. He does not take any medications on a regular basis. He is allergic to penicillin, which causes a rash. He is married, has two children, and is employed full-time in computer sales. He denies any tobacco use; drinks "a few beers a week," and denies recreational drug use.

Example 1–2 is longer than Example 1–1. It is also more thorough and complete and helps answer the questions a reader would not have been able to answer after reading Example 1–1. Example 1–2 does a better job of documenting aggravating and alleviating factors and pertinent positives and negatives. Notice also the use of quotation marks to indicate a verbatim response from the patient. There will be times when you want to include the patient's exact words in your documentation. Worksheet 1–1, at the end of this chapter, will help you identify and organize subjective information. Worksheet 1–2 will give you additional practice using the abbreviations that are presented in this chapter.

MEDICOLEGAL ALERT!

When a condition or symptom involves anything that is symmetrical, specify the area of concern and do so consistently. In Example 1–2, the patient complained of left knee pain. Always check that you document left knee when you are referring to history and report left knee findings from the physical examination. Most conditions involving the left extremity warrant examination of and comparison to the right extremity. Even one discrepancy in use of left or right could raise doubts as to which area is being examined or treated. Malpractice lawyers will look for such discrepancies and will be sure to point them out, which might damage your credibility.

Chapter Summary

- Subjective is what the subject tells you.
- This information is often referred to as the patient's history.
- Physical examination findings are not subjective, but are objective.
- When documenting, put all pertinent positives together, then the pertinent negatives. This makes it easier to keep the information in a logical format.
- Use quotation marks to identify the patient's exact words.
- Remember, if it is not documented, it was not done!

Part A

A patient presents with a chief complaint of back pain. Below are several statements from the HPI for a chief complaint of back pain. Number them in the order they should appear in the subjective paragraph.

1. _____ Pertinent negative associated symptom: The patient denies any trauma.

2. _____ Aggravating factor: The pain is worse after standing or walking for more than 20 minutes.

3. _____ Onset: The pain started three days ago after moving some heavy furniture.

4. _____ Pertinent positive associated symptom: The patient has had a tingling sensation in the right buttock area.

5. _____ Severity: The pain is described as a dull ache and is rated as a 4/10.

Part B

After the HPI, the past medical history (PMH) should be documented. Place a check beside all statements that are part of the PMH.

_____ There is no family history of heart disease.   _____ The patient smokes 1 pack per day.

_____ The patient is allergic to penicillin.   _____ The patient works as a mechanic.

_____ No chronic medical conditions.   _____ The patient takes Zantac daily.

Part C

Which of the following would be documented as subjective information? Circle all that apply.

vital signs   family history   onset of chief complaint

history obtained from spouse   complete blood count (CBC) results

medications   physical examination findings

information from previous   review of systems
  medical records

X-ray report

These abbreviations were introduced in Chapter 1. Beside each, write its meaning.

S _____

O _____

A _____

P _____

CC _____

HPI _____

PMH _____

ROS _____

CBC _____

FH _____

SH _____

See Appendix B for answers to these worksheets.

Chapter 2

Objective

Objective information is what you can see or observe first-hand. Primarily, objective data are vital signs (VS), physical examination findings, and results from laboratory or diagnostic studies. All physical examination findings are documented together followed by results of laboratory tests or other diagnostic tests. The interpretation of an electrocardiogram (ECG or EKG), for instance, is objective data. You should always document if the interpretation of a study or test is your own or is made by someone else.

Formats for Documenting Objective Information

Two formats are commonly used for documenting the objective information portion of a SOAP note. Example 2–1 shows the narrative paragraph, and Example 2–2 shows the system heading format. Either format is acceptable. Some healthcare providers prefer the system heading format because the use of headings makes it easier to find specific information. Instead of reading the entire objective section, a reader can go quickly and easily to the system related to the chief complaint. As you perform the physical examination in a head-to-toe fashion, your documentation should proceed just as regularly. Figure 2–1 shows the usual order of documenting the physical examination. The objective section will also have pertinent positives and negatives, and again we recommend that you list all positives together, and then list the negatives. This provides a more logical flow when reading the entry. If examina-

tion of a specific system is not indicated, based on the subjective information you elicited, omit that heading from the list. It is not necessary to list each system of the body and then put "not examined" or "not applicable". Worksheet 2.1 at the end of this chapter will help you organize subjective and objective information.

EXAMPLE 2–1
NARRATIVE FORMAT

The patient is a 6-year-old Hispanic female who is alert and cooperative. Her temperature is 99.2, respirations 20, pulse is 88, and blood pressure (BP) is 96/60. Her skin is dry and intact without any rashes or lesions. The turgor is good. The head is normocephalic and atraumatic. The pupils are equal, round, and reactive to light. The tympanic membranes are intact bilaterally without erythema or effusion. Cone of light and bony landmarks are visible bilaterally. The ear canals are without swelling or discharge. The nose is patent without any rhinorrhea. Oropharynx is without erythema or exudates, and the mucous membranes are moist and intact. The neck is supple without any lymphadenopathy. The breath sounds are clear to auscultation without any adventitious sounds. Heart is regular rate and rhythm without murmur. The chest wall is nontender and there are no sternal retractions. The abdomen is soft and nondistended. The bowel sounds are physiologic in all four quadrants. There is no organomegaly and no masses are palpated. The extremities show full range of motion of all joints, and there is no clubbing, cyanosis, or edema. Cranial nerves II–XII are grossly intact, and there are no focal neurological deficits.

EXAMPLE 2–2
SYSTEMS HEADINGS FORMAT

General: The patient is a 6-year-old Hispanic female who is alert and cooperative. Her temperature is 99.2, respirations 20, pulse is 88, and BP is 96/60.

Skin: dry and intact without any rashes or lesions. The turgor is good.

HEENT (head, eyes, ears, nose, and throat): The head is normocephalic and atraumatic. The pupils are equal, round, and reactive to light. The tympanic membranes are intact bilaterally without erythema or effusion. Cone of light and bony landmarks are visible bilaterally. The ear canals are without swelling or discharge. The nose is patent without any rhinorrhea. Oropharynx is without erythema or exudates, and the mucous membranes are moist and intact.

Neck: The neck is supple without any lymphadenopathy.

Chest: The breath sounds are clear to auscultation without any adventitious sounds. Heart is regular rate and rhythm without murmur. The chest wall is nontender and there are no sternal retractions.

Abdomen: soft and nondistended. The bowel sounds are physiologic in all four quadrants. There is no organomegaly and no masses are palpated.

Extremities: full range of motion of all joints, and there is no clubbing, cyanosis or edema.

Neurological: Cranial nerves II-XII are grossly intact and there are no focal neurological deficits.

Objective Versus Subjective Information

One of the most common mistakes made when documenting objective information is to include subjective information. It can be difficult to remember which is which. If a patient tells you she has pain in her foot, that is subjective information because it is history information the patient has provided. If you palpate the patient's foot, and she reacts with grimacing, withdrawing the foot, or vocalizing pain, that is objective information because you were able to observe her reaction to the palpation. Ask yourself "Is this something I could observe, or is this something the patient would tell me?"

Application Exercise 2.1

Look at the following information, and indicate which is subjective (S) or objective (O).
____ The right hand is swollen.
____ There is no tenderness to palpation of the right knee.
____ My left arm feels numb and has a tingling sensation.
____ Patient is hard of hearing.
____ No respiratory distress is noted.
____ Patient denies allergies to any medication.

General information (patient identifier such as gender, age, and race)

Vital signs, height and weight, very brief mental status description

Skin

HEENT

Neck

Chest (including lungs)

Cardiovascular

Abdomen

Genitourinary

Musculoskeletal

Neurological

Figure 2–1. Suggested order of documenting a physical examination.

APPLICATION EXERCISE 2.1 ANSWERS

Look at the following information, and indicate which is subjective (S) or objective (O).

_O_ The right hand is swollen.

_O_ There is no tenderness to palpation of the right knee.

_S_ My left arm feels numb and has a tingling sensation.

_O_ Patient is hard of hearing.

_O_ No respiratory distress is noted.

_S_ Patient denies allergies to any medication.

Refer to Worksheet 2.2 at the end of this chapter to compare subjective and objective information, and complete the worksheet as instructed.

Documenting Diagnostic Test Results

Results of laboratory and other diagnostic tests, such as radiographs, are objective findings. These should be documented after all the information from the physical examination has been documented. Give the name of the test first, then the result (i.e., CBC shows a white blood cell count [WBC] of 5.8, hemoglobin [Hgb] of 11, and hematocrit [Hct] of 34). If all the results are within normal limits, you may document as "the CBC is within normal limits (WNL)." If one component of a panel of tests is abnormal, but the rest are normal, you could document "the comprehensive metabolic panel (CMP) shows a potassium of 5.2; otherwise, the results are WNL."

▼ MEDICOLEGAL ALERT!

Failure to follow up on abnormal laboratory test or studies can be a component of alleged malpractice. Every office should have a protocol for tracking laboratory results as they come in to the office. You must notify the patient of any abnormal test results and have a follow-up plan to determine why the results are abnormal. Failure to recognize that there is an abnormal test result, or failure to follow-up on an abnormal test result could have disastrous results.

If you plan to order diagnostic tests but do not have the results at the time you are document-

ing, this is usually referred to as part of the plan instead of objective "finding". This is because there are no results to observe yet. Consider the scenario of a 17-year-old patient who presents with right ankle pain. After gathering all the history, or subjective information, you perform the physical examination, or the objective information. You decide to order an x-ray of the ankle. If you cannot perform the x-ray on-site, the patient will have to go to an outpatient facility for that x-ray. Dr Jones, the radiologist at the facility, typically phones you immediately with the results of the x-ray, so you ask the patient to return to your office after the x-ray is taken. When you get the results, you would document "x-ray of the right ankle is negative for any fracture or other acute findings per Dr. Jones." If you can perform x-rays on site, or if the patient returns with x-rays from the other facility, you would interpret them, and document your findings as your own (i.e., I did not see any fracture or other acute findings on the x-ray of the right ankle).

Interventions Done During the Visit

Interventions done during the visit are also documented as part of the objective section. Suppose the patient described above with the ankle pain is seen at 5:30 p.m. You cannot do x-rays on site, and the outpatient facility where he would have an x-ray done is closed for the day. In the meantime, you apply a posterior splint and instruct the patient on crutch-walking. These interventions are documented in the objective section of the note. Obtaining an x-ray is part of your plan, which will be discussed further in Chapter 4. If the patient were instructed to return tomorrow after x-rays have been taken, that would be documented as part of the plan.

Worksheet 2–3 at the end of this chapter will give you additional practice using the abbreviations that were presented in this chapter.

Chapter Summary

- Objective is what you observe. Others should be able to observe the same thing for it to be objective.

- When documenting physical examination findings, you can use either the narrative format or a systems heading format.
- List pertinent positive findings together first, then pertinent negatives.
- If a system is not examined, do not include the heading for that system.
- Results of laboratory, other diagnostic studies, and interventions done during the visit should be documented in the objective section following physical examination findings, as a continuation of the paragraph or under a separate heading.

- Remember, if it is not documented, it was not done!

Organizing Subjective and Objective Information

Part A

Number the following sentences in the order they should appear in the subjective paragraph.

1. _____ Onset: The symptoms started 3 days ago.

2. _____ Pertinent positive associated signs and symptoms: The patient has had cough and low-grade fever.

3. _____ Aggravating/alleviating factors: Over the counter cough medication has not decreased his cough.

4. _____ Chief complaint: The patient complains of cold symptoms.

5. _____ Pertinent negative associated signs and symptoms: The patient has not had increased sputum production or shortness of breath.

Part B

Number the following sentences in the order they should appear in the objective paragraph, according to "head-to-toe" order.

1. _____ The abdomen is soft and nondistended.

2. _____ The oropharynx shows some erythema of the posterior pharyngeal wall but no exudates.

3. _____ Auscultation of the lungs does not reveal any adventitious breath sounds.

4. _____ The neck is supple with full range of motion and there are no signs of meningeal irritation.

5. _____ The skin is warm to touch and without cyanosis.

Identifying Subjective and Objective Data

Read the following sentences, and determine if the information is subjective (S) or objective (O).

1. _____ On a scale of 1–10, the pain is a 7.

2. _____ Bruising is seen at the lateral border of the foot.

3. _____ The patient denies any swelling of the wrist.

4. _____ There is tenderness to palpation over the maxillary sinuses.

5. _____ The patient walks with a limp.

6. _____ Weakness of the left arm is noted when compared to the right arm.

7. _____ The patient noticed a rash on his leg 2 days ago.

8. _____ I interpret the ECG as showing ischemic changes.

9. _____ The radiology report indicates that the computed tomography (CT) scan is normal.

10. _____ The patient denies shortness of breath.

11. _____ "My left arm feels numb."

12. _____ The patient is alert and oriented.

13. _____ Nasal flaring is noted.

14. _____ The nurse reports that the patient refused his medications this morning.

15. _____ An allergy to penicillin is documented in the patient's chart.

16. _____ Grip with the right hand is weaker than the left.

17. _____ The patient complains of a ringing sensation in the right ear.

18. _____ The patient complains of pain over the sinus area of the forehead.

19. _____ The patient is a 7-year-old well developed, well nourished Asian-American child, who is alert and oriented.

20. _____ The patient said she felt warm at home, as if she had a fever.

These abbreviations were introduced in Chapter 2. Beside each, write its meaning.

ECG, EKG _____

BP _____

HEENT _____

WBC _____

WNL _____

CMP _____

CT _____

VS _____

Hct _____

Hgb _____

See Appendix B for the answers to these worksheets.

Assessment

$\mathcal{N}$ ow that you have taken the history and performed the physical examination, it is time to assess the patient's condition. The assessment is the diagnosis, your impression of the patient's condition. It is based on your analysis of the patient's history, physical examination findings, and the results of any tests you have at the time. If you are not sure of the diagnosis, you may use a presumptive diagnosis, such as a symptom, complaint, condition, or problem.

EXAMPLE 3–1

Diagnosis	Urinary tract infection (UTI)
Symptom	Dysuria
Complaint	Abdominal pain, suprapubic
Condition	Diabetes mellitus
Problem	Hearing loss

The Differential Diagnoses

When a definitive diagnosis is not available, it is helpful to think of, and perhaps write down, the differential diagnoses (DDX). The differential diagnoses are a list of possible conditions the patient might have that have not yet been ruled in or out and that may require further work-up. It is similar to a worksheet, allowing you to prioritize your plan of care.

When listing the differential diagnoses, list in order of most likely to least likely. The list should not be all-inclusive but a result of critically analyzing the available data. The DDX guides you through the diagnostic work-up and the treatment plan. It also lets other readers understand your reasoning and supports your plan of action.

Developing the Differential Diagnoses

Once you have ascertained the chief complaint, you immediately begin formulating a list of possible causes. As you proceed with obtaining the history and performing the physical examination, you are continuously analyzing data to narrow the DDX. Some facilities will have laboratory and x-ray services readily available, enabling you to make a definitive diagnosis. When these are not available, order them in the plan section of your SOAP note.

Consider the following comprehensive example.

EXAMPLE 3–2

S: Mr. Jensen is a 67-year-old Caucasian male who presents with a chief complaint of tiredness and "feeling weak" for the past 6 or 7 months. Before this, he was in his usual state of good health. He became concerned about 2 weeks ago when he started feeling "winded" toward the end of his usual two-mile walk, which he is able to complete. He denies shortness of breath, dyspnea, chest pain, or claudication. He notes that his energy level has decreased and feels like he is "losing strength." Taking a multivitamin has not improved his symptoms.

Medical: hypertension (HTN) for 8 years; hypercholesterolemia for 3 years.

Surgical: left inguinal hernia repair, 1995; repair of torn right rotator cuff, 1987.

No blood transfusions.

Current medications: Cardizem 120 milligrams (mg) SR qd, Mevacor 20 mg qd, Centrum

(Continued)

EXAMPLE 3–2 *(Continued)*

Silver multivitamin qd. Acetaminophen as required (PRN). Maalox PRN.

Allergies: SULFA causes a systemic rash.

Immunizations: Tetanus and pneumovax 2 years ago. Flu shot last fall. Childhood chickenpox.

Health maintenance: Last physical 2 years ago. Cholesterol was around 185. BP has been stable for the past 7 years.

FAMILY HX (History):

Father is deceased, age 74, complications of chronic obstructive pulmonary disease (COPD) and alcoholism. Mother deceased, age 70, breast cancer. Brother, age 69, has HTN. Brother, deceased at age 20 from combat head wound. Three children, alive and well. Negative family history for diabetes, myocardial infarction. Positive family history of cancer, hypertension/coronary artery disease (CAD), and COPD.

SOCIAL HX:

Mr. Jensen is a retired electrician. He is married and lives in a single story home with his wife. They have three adult children who all live nearby. He smokes a pipe about three times a week. He denies any alcohol or recreational drug use. He is still active and walks approximately 2 miles 4 out of 7 days per week. He also rides a bicycle occasionally.

REVIEW OF SYSTEMS:

General: easily fatigued, feels weak. Denies fever, chills, night sweats, or weight loss.

HEENT: He has worn glasses since 1985; last eye examination 3 months ago. Denies loss of vision, double vision, or history of cataracts. Denies any change in hearing, smell, taste. Denies pain or discomfort in ears, eyes, nose, throat or sinuses, nasal discharge, change in voice.

Neck: Denies swollen glands or other areas of swelling, or restriction of movement.

Respiratory: As above, feels "winded" toward the end of his two-mile walk. Has an occasional morning cough that is nonproductive. Denies shortness of breath (SOB), dyspnea on exertion (DOE), hemoptysis.

Cardiovascular: Denies chest pain with or without exertion, orthopnea, palpitations, irregularities in rhythm, chest wall pain, venous distention, swelling of hands or feet.

GI: "Indigestion" occurs no more than two or three times a week and is always relieved with antacids. Denies any change in bowel habits, melena, hematochezia, change in appetite, nausea, vomiting, diarrhea, constipation, cramping, bloating, difficulty swallowing, hemorrhoids.

GU: Denies dysuria, hesitancy, frequency, hematuria, penile discharge, scrotal or testicular masses, history of sexually transmitted disease (STD).

Musculoskeletal: Denies joint swelling, pain, redness, decreased range of motion (ROM); neck, back, or extremity pain.

Neurological: Denies near-syncope, dizziness, persistent or uncharacteristic headaches, abnormal gait.

Hematological: Denies easy bruising, prolonged or abnormal bleeding, delayed wound healing, or recurrent infections.

Psychiatric: Denies depressed mood, anxiety, sleep disturbances, suicidal ideations, hallucinations, delusions, or history of affective or personality disorders.

O: BP 134/80; P 82 and regular; R 16 and regular; Temperature 97.8 orally; Wt 174 lb; Ht 70"

General: Mr. Jensen is a well-developed, well-nourished (WDWN) Caucasian male who is in no acute distress (NAD). He is alert and oriented (A&O) × 3

Skin: no rashes, cyanosis, or jaundice.

HEENT:

Head normocephalic, atraumatic. No scleral icteris. Pupils equally round and reactive to light and accommodation. Wearing glasses. Canals are clear without erythema, swelling, or discharge. Tympanic membranes (TMs) intact, pearly gray, with normal cone of light. Nose patent bilaterally without deformity or discharge. Oropharynx without erythema or exudate. No mucosal lesions. Wearing well-fitting upper and lower dentures in good repair.

NECK:

Supple, nontender, full ROM. No adenopathy or masses palpated. No tracheal deviation, thyromegaly, or carotid bruits.

CHEST:

Breath sounds clear to auscultation in all lung fields. Respiratory excursion symmetrical. Heart with regular rate and rhythm. No murmurs, gallops, or rubs. Point of maximum impulse (PMI) normal without thrills or heaves. Chest wall is nontender to palpation.

ABDOMEN:

Soft, nontender. No masses or organomegaly. Normoactive bowel sounds in all four quadrants. No guarding or rebound noted.

RECTAL/GU:

Prostate: normal size, nontender, and without masses. Formed, brown stool guaiac POSITIVE. No rectal masses. Circumcised male, without testicular or scrotal masses or tenderness. No penile lesions or discharge. No hernia. Well-healed surgical scar left inguinal area. No inguinal adenopathy.

(Continued)

Chapter 3 **Assessment** 23

EXAMPLE 3–2 (Continued)

MUSCULOSKELETAL:

No deformities, joint effusions, clubbing, cyanosis, or edema. Full ROM of all four extremities and back. Well-healed surgical scar over the right anterior shoulder.

NEUROLOGICAL:

Cranial nerve (CN) II-XII grossly intact. Motor: +5/5 upper and lower extremities. Sensory intact to pinprick. Deep tendon reflexes (DTRs) intact and symmetrical. Mood and affect appropriate.

A: 1) Fatigue
   DDX: secondary to #2; anemia
   2) Hemoccult positive stool
   DDX: r/o colon cancer; gastric/duodenal ulcer; polyps
   3) Hypertension – stable
   4) Hypercholesterolemia

Read the following note, and answer the questions.

Application Exercise 3.1

S: Ms. Kearns is a 42-year-old woman who presents with a CC of chest pain × 3 days.

1. List your DDX based on the CC:

_____

_____

_____

S: It started yesterday, approximately 2 hours after she had "vigorously" cleaned her bathroom using a new cleaner, then worsened while she was gardening later in the day. Initially, the pain started in the middle of her chest. Today it radiates to the left anterior chest area. At rest, the pain is described as an "aching," with a pain scale rating of 2/10; however, with moving about and taking a deep breath, the pain becomes sharp and shooting with a rating of 7/10. She feels slightly feverish; has a dry, non-productive cough; is slightly short of breath at rest, which worsens with activity; has a clear runny nose, and a slight frontal headache. The chest pain does not radiate to her arm, neck, or jaw. She denies sore throat, ear pain, nausea, vomiting, abdominal or back pain. Advil, 2 tablets every 8 hours, seems to help a little. No relief of cough with Robitussin DM. PMH: positive for allergic rhinitis, appendectomy, and tonsillectomy. Current medications: Allegra 180

mg/d PRN allergies. No known drug allergies (NKDA). FH: no cardiopulmonary diseases or cancer. She has smoked 1 pack per day (PPD) for the past 15 years.

2. Based on the patient's subjective information, has your DDX changed? If so, list your revised DDX:

_____

_____

_____

O: VS: 144/90, T 99.4 orally; P 98; R 22; Ht 5′6″; Wt 150 lb
This 42-year-old black woman appears mildly anxious but in no acute distress. She is A&O × 3.
Skin: no rashes or cyanosis.

HEENT:

TMs are unremarkable. Nose is slightly congested with pink turbinates and clear discharge. Mild pharyngeal erythema without exudates.

NECK:

Supple, nontender. No adenopathy, thyromegaly, or jugular venous distention (JVD) noted.

CHEST:

Breath sounds are clear. No wheezes on forced expiration, adventitious sounds, rubs, or dullness to percussion. Chest wall is tender to palpation in the left, 4th to 7th costochondral area.

Heart: heart rate (HR) 98 and regular without murmurs or gallop. Normal S1 and S2.

ABDOMEN:

Soft, nontender. No rebound, guarding, masses, or hepatosplenomegaly (HSM). Bowel sounds are normoactive.

3. If you do not have a definitive diagnosis, list up to 3 DDX:

_____

_____

_____

4. What diagnostic testing, if any, would you order to further narrow the DDX?

_____

_____

5. Based on all the information available, what is your assessment?

Copyright © 2004 by F.A. Davis Company. All rights reserved.

Notice how your differential diagnoses are modified by various factors such as age, vital signs, and the presence or absence of a previous history of cardiopulmonary, GI, MS, emotional, or other diseases that can cause chest pain. The subjective and objective information will help you narrow the DDX to the most likely diagnosis. Appropriate diagnostic tests can also help further refine the DDX. If you do not have a definitive diagnosis when the patient leaves your facility, you can use "Chest Pain" as the assessment.

APPLICATION EXERCISE 3.1 ANSWERS

1. What is your DDX based on the CC?
Skin: herpes zoster
Heart: angina, myocardial infarction (MI), endocarditis, pericardial effusion
Respiratory: bronchitis, pneumonia, pleurisy
GI: gastric/duodenal ulcer, gastroesophageal reflux disease (GERD), hiatal hernia
MS: costochondritis, chest wall strain/sprain
Neuro: anxiety disorder
Breast: fibrocystic breast disease, cancer, mastitis

2. Based on the patient's subjective information, has your DDX changed? If so, list your revised DDX:
More likely: pleurisy, pneumonia, costochondritis, chest wall strain/sprain, endocarditis.
Less likely: angina, MI, breast or GI etiology, zoster, bronchitis. Would add COPD and lung cancer.

3. If you do not have a definitive diagnosis, list 3 DDX.
Costochondritis, pleurisy, rule out (r/o) pneumonia

4. What diagnostic testing, if any, would you order to further narrow the DDX?
CBC, posteroanterior (PA) and lateral chest x-ray (CXR), EKG. Consider spirometry.
Here are the results of your tests:
CBC: WBC 7.0 with normal differential; the remainder is WNL. CXR: normal, per radiologist.
EKG: normal sinus rhythm without acute changes, per my interpretation.
Spirometry: normal.

5. Based on all the information available, what is your assessment?

Costochondritis
For further practice, see Worksheet 3.1 at the end of this chapter.

Assessment and ICD-10-CM Coding

ICD-10-CM stands for International Classification of Diseases (ICD)-Tenth Edition-Clinical Modification. Published annually by the U.S. Public Health Service and the Centers for Medicare and Medicaid Services (CMMS), it is the standardized system for applying a numeric code to each diagnosis. These codes are generally used to determine the level of reimbursement for medical services rendered. They are also used by outside agencies and organizations to forecast healthcare needs, evaluate facilities and services, review costs, and conduct studies of trends in diseases over the years. The medical community and the insurance industry have procedures and rules to facilitate the processing of claims. Coding is one such procedure. Medical record documentation is another. Specially trained personnel generally assign a code utilizing data from the medical record. The medical record must include documentation that supports the assessment. The quality and accuracy of your medical records is vital to the reimbursement process, which in turn is vital to the delivery of health care. You must write your notes in a clear, concise, and legible manner using a standard format.

MEDICOLEGAL ALERT!
Although getting paid is a very important issue for physicians' offices, they should never code for reimbursement purposes only. This can be construed as fraud. Remember, your documentation must support the diagnoses reported.

Some Coding Rules

The rules of coding can guide practitioners into developing good documentation skills. Here are a few of the rules:

1. The codes used must justify any tests ordered.
   • If a urine pregnancy test is performed in the office, then a reason for obtaining that test must be included in the codes for that office visit. The diagnosis may be amenorrhea

(626.0), menometrorrhagia (626.2), or galact-orrhea (676.6).

2. Assign an ICD-10 code that reflects the most specific diagnosis that is known at the time.
   • The patient's diagnosis is gastroenteritis (558.9). If you know, with reasonable certainty, that it is viral, then use the code for viral gastroenteritis, 008.8. Suppose that the patient's original complaint was diarrhea (787.91). You order a stool culture and it comes back positive for shigella. When the patient returns for a follow-up visit, the diagnosis would then be enteritis, shigella (004.9).

3. The first diagnosis should reflect the patient's CC or why they sought medical attention.
   • Let's say that the patient's diagnoses for this office visit are abdominal pain, depression, and diabetes mellitus. The patient came in because of abdominal pain. This would be the first diagnosis listed.

4. Code a chronic condition as often as applicable to the patient's condition.
   • Using the preceding example, diabetes mellitus is a chronic condition that may be related to, or cause, the abdominal pain. Listing it in the assessment portion of your notes points this fact out.

5. Code all documented conditions that coexist at the time of the visit.
   • Depression is a coexisting condition that may alter the patient's perception of the abdominal pain. He could be thinking the pain signifies cancer. He may be taking antidepressant medication, which could cause the pain. Adding chronic and coexisting conditions to the assessment summarizes the scope of the patient's problem to you and other readers.

6. Do not use "rule out…" as a diagnosis.
   • There is no code for this. Instead, use a symptom, complaint, condition or problem. You may use "rule out" in your DDX to guide you in your plan of care, although it is not necessary.

Nomenclature for Diagnoses

Diagnostic terminology can be broad or specific. It is preferable to be as descriptive as the data allows. Consider the following examples.

EXAMPLE 3–3

BROAD	SPECIFIC
neck pain	acute cervical sprain
upper respiratory infection (URI)	allergic rhinitis
chest pain	costochondritis; pleurisy
cough	pneumonia; COPD
arthralgia	osteoarthritis; rheumatoid arthritis

In general, you should use the medical term for a diagnosis, symptom, complaint, or problem. Instead of "runny nose" you would use "rhinorrhea." This does not work in every situation. There is no medical term for "chest pain" when used as a diagnosis, unless you know what is causing the chest pain. For more practice using medical terminology and abbreviations see Worksheets 3.2 and 3.3 at the end of this chapter.

EXAMPLE 3–4

Instead of:		Use:	
	joint pains		arthralgias
	difficulty swallowing		dysphagia
	menstrual cramps		dysmenorrhea
	blood in urine		hematuria
	yeast infection		candidiasis

Chapter Summary

• Assessment is the same as diagnosis.
• If a definitive diagnosis is not apparent, a symptom, complaint, condition or problem may be used.
• The differential diagnoses are a list of possible diagnoses to be considered
• Further diagnostic testing may be needed to narrow the differential diagnoses, enabling you to make a definitive diagnosis.
• The medical record must include documentation that supports the assessment, which is assigned a code for billing purposes.
• Do not use "rule out …" as a diagnosis.
• Use appropriate medical terms.
• Remember, if it is not documented, it was not done!

S: This 6-year-old child presents with a sore throat times 3 days. His mother states that he has had a fever of 101.5 orally, seems to have difficulty swallowing, and complains of a headache. His appetite is decreased. He has a runny nose with clear discharge. Denies cough, abdominal pain, vomiting, or diarrhea. There are no known exposures to communicable diseases. Tylenol helps the fever and sore throat "a little." PMH is negative. Meds: none. NKDA. The child is generally healthy.

O: T 100.8 (oral), P 98, R 20, BP 100/64

General: WDWN Caucasian male in NAD.

Skin: no rash

HEENT:

Canals and TMs are unremarkable. Nasal mucosa is slightly congested with pink turbinates and clear discharge. Pharynx shows 3+ injected tonsils with scant exudates.

NECK:

Supple. Tender, moderately enlarged tonsillar lymph nodes.

HEART:

Rate 98 and regular without murmur.

LUNGS:

Clear to auscultation. No adventitious sounds. Nonlabored breathing.

Abdomen: Soft, nondistended. Mildly tender throughout without guarding, rebound, or change in facial expression. No organomegaly or masses. Bowel sounds are normoactive.

1. What is your assessment of the patient described in the preceding example?

_____

_____

2. What else would you include in your differential diagnoses?

_____

_____

3. What tests, if any, would you order?

_____

_____

Fill in the blanks using correct medical terminology for the lay terms on the left.

1. miscarriage   _____

2. mole   _____

3. nearsightedness   _____

4. stiff neck   _____

5. athlete's foot   _____

6. hives   _____

7. rubeola (measles)   _____

8. tingling   _____

9. loss of appetite   _____

10. fear of crowds   _____

11. canker sore   _____

12. navel   _____

These abbreviations were introduced in Chapter 3. Beside each, write its meaning.

UTI	_____	GI	_____
DDX	_____	A&O	_____
PRN	_____	URI	_____
COPD	_____	CMMS	_____
CAD	_____	d	_____
HX, Hx	_____	DM	_____
SOB	_____	GERD	_____
DOE	_____	GU	_____
STDs	_____	Ht	_____
ROM	_____	HTN	_____
WDWN	_____	mg	_____
NAD	_____	MI	_____
TMs	_____	MS	_____
PMI	_____	P	_____
CN	_____	PA	_____
DTRs	_____	PPD	_____
NKDA	_____	q	_____
JVD	_____	R	_____
HR	_____	R/O	_____
HSM	_____	T	_____
CXR	_____	Wt	_____
ICD-10	_____		

See Appendix B for answers to these worksheets.

Chapter 4

Plan

$\mathcal{T}$his section of the SOAP note is where you establish your plan of care. Each diagnosis in the assessment must be addressed in the plan. The items in the plan should be documented in an orderly manner, which may vary depending on your practice setting. One suggested format is the following:

1. Tests and referrals: any diagnostic tests, such as laboratory tests and x-rays, and referrals to specialists, therapists (physical, occupational), counselors, etc.

2. Pharmaceutical: prescriptions and over-the-counter medication recommendations.

3. Patient education: explanations and advice given to patients and family members.

4. Follow-up instructions: when the patient is to return, the conditions or symptoms that indicate the patient should return sooner, and when to go to another facility such as an emergency department or urgent care center.

Refer to Ms. Kearns from Chapter 3, Application Exercise 3.1

Application Exercise 4.1

Assume that your facility does not have the capability to perform any diagnostic testing. The assessment is "chest pain." Write your plan using the SOAP format.

_____

_____

_____

_____

Compare your plan with the following answer.

APPLICATION EXERCISE 4.1 ANSWERS

A: CHEST PAIN

P: CBC

PA & LATERAL CXR.

EKG

BIAXIN XL 500 MG, ONE PO BID, PC #20, NO REFILLS.

IBUPROFEN 800 MG ONE EVERY 6–8 HRS, PC, PRN PAIN. #40, ONE REFILL.

STRETCHING EXERCISES Q 2 HOURS WHILE AWAKE; HANDOUT PROVIDED.

DISCUSSED POSSIBLE CAUSES OF CHEST PAIN WITH PATIENT.

FOLLOW-UP IN 2 DAYS. RETURN SOONER, OR GO TO ED, PRN WORSENING OF SOB OR CHEST PAIN.

Application Exercise 4.2

Ms. Kearns returns for a follow-up visit 2 days later. Refer to her test results in Application

Exercise 3–1, answer number 5. The assessment is "costochondritis." Write your plan.

_____

_____

_____

_____

_____

Compare your plan with the answer below.

APPLICATION EXERCISE 4.2 ANSWERS

A: COSTOCHONDRITIS

P: DISCONTINUE (D/C) BIAXIN.

CONTINUE IBUPROFEN PRN PAIN.

CONTINUE STRETCHING EXERCISES.

AVOID LIFTING GREATER THAN 20 POUNDS OR EXCESSIVE USE OF ARMS UNTIL PAIN HAS RESOLVED. _____

RETURN TO CLINIC (RTC) PRN SYMPTOMS WORSEN OR DO NOT IMPROVE AFTER 1 WEEK.

Alternate Format for Plan Section

One variation of the SOAP note format is to list the plan components under each diagnosis, instead of in a separate plan section. The following examples illustrate the difference. Refer to Mr. Jensen's note in Chapter 3, Example 3–2.

EXAMPLE 4–1

Typical SOAP note format:
A: 1) Fatigue
        DDX: secondary to #2; anemia
    2) Hemoccult positive stool
        DDX: rule out (R/O) colon cancer; gastric/duodenal ulcer; polyps
    3) Hypertension: stable
    4) Hypercholesterolemia
P: Check CBC.
    Continue same meds.
    May continue Maalox and acetaminophen PRN.
    Refer to GI: Michael Bennett, MD.

Discussed possible causes for hemoccult positive stool with patient.
Follow-up after GI consult.
RTC or go to ED PRN dizziness, feeling faint, abdominal pain, or vomiting.

EXAMPLE 4–2

Combining Assessment and Plan into one section:
Assessment and Plan:
    1) Fatigue
        DDX: secondary to #2; anemia
        Check CBC
    2) Hemoccult positive stool
        DDX: r/o colon cancer; gastric/duodenal ulcer; polyps
        Refer to GI: Michael Bennett, MD
        Discussed possible causes of hemoccult positive stool with patient.
        Follow-up after GI consult.
        RTC or go to ED PRN dizziness, feeling faint, abdominal pain, or vomiting.
    3) Hypertension – stable
        Continue Cardizem SR 120 mg qd.
    4) Hypercholesterolemia
        Continue Mevacor 20 mg qd.

Patient Education

Patient education is considered by many to be a cornerstone of the physician assistant (PA) profession. When a patient has a positive encounter with a healthcare provider, it is often because "the provider took time to explain everything." Educating patients about their condition or disease enables them to take control of their health. Patients should be encouraged to be active participants in their own healthcare, rather than to take a passive role, which may improve compliance with treatment. Figure 4–1 is one example of a patient education handout.

Most patients want to know what is causing their symptoms, what their treatment options are, the expected outcome, and why or when to return to the office, e.g., signs that they are not getting better or that their condition is worsening. When medication is prescribed or recommended, they need to know what the benefits and the risks are, among many other details (see Chapter 12).

Follow-up visits are an opportune time to ask patients if they have any questions about what was discussed previously. Encouragement and reinforcement will promote patient understanding, which, in turn, may lead to a more favorable outcome.

▼
MEDICOLEGAL ALERT!

Documentation of patient education is not only good medical practice, it may prevent a lawsuit. Remember: if it is not documented, it was not done! This applies to medications prescribed, tests performed, consents obtained, warnings, recommendations, patient education, and follow-up instructions.

Printed handouts are a valuable tool to reinforce what you have told patients. There are many resources available on just about any topic you may encounter. Some books have tear-out sheets to give to patients. Others have pages you can photocopy. There are software programs and websites that allow you to customize and personalize handouts with your office logo and information. Pharmaceutical companies often have patient education information relating to their products; i.e., Lilly makes Humalog insulin and can provide diabetic diets, logbooks for patients to record blood sugar readings, and educational materials on diabetes for patients and their families. When you document what handouts and materials you gave the patient, this will remind you to inquire about the patient's understanding of the material at the next follow-up visit. Simply giving the patient printed material does not meet your obligation to provide patient education. You should determine if they read and understood the material and if they have any questions about what they read.

Follow-Up Instructions

It is important to document follow-up instructions at each patient visit, regardless of what the visit was for. "RTC PRN" is not specific enough. Instead, give more specific instructions, such as "RTC PRN symptoms worsen or do not improve after 3 days." Give a specific period for the patient's condition to improve.

Follow-Up Instructions for Illnesses

If a patient has been taking antibiotics for an ear infection and has not improved after 3 days, the patient may need a different one. Think of potential complications that could occur, such as acute mastoiditis, labyrinthitis, or meningitis. Document the specific symptoms that should prompt follow-up, such as persistent fever, headache, dizziness, nausea and vomiting, and neck stiffness. This is especially important in pediatrics and in situations where the patient's condition could deteriorate rapidly. For example, a patient presents complaining of headache, fever, and myalgias for the past 2 days. Your assessment is influenza, but there are other more serious conditions that would be in the DDX. The patient needs to be reevaluated if the condition changes, so you instruct the patient to notify you immediately or to go to the emergency department if vomiting, neck stiffness, or worsening of the headache occurs. Failure to document your instructions to the patient is considered failure to provide these instructions.

For further reinforcement of what was covered in this chapter, see Worksheets 4.1 and 4.2 at the end of this chapter.

Chapter Summary

- The Plan section is where you establish your plan of care.
- Components of the plan include tests and referrals, pharmacological therapy, patient education, and follow-up instructions.
- Patient education is considered by many to be a cornerstone of the PA profession.
- Documentation of patient education may prevent a lawsuit.
- Printed handouts are a valuable tool and help reinforce what you have told the patient.
- Give a specific time frame for the patient's condition to improve or for when the patient should be re-evaluated if no improvement.

- Remember, if it is not documented, it was not done!

Sleep Hygiene Guide

- Take a hot bath to raise your temperature for 30 minutes within 2 hours of bedtime. A hot drink may also help you to relax.

- Daily exercise at least 6 hours before bedtime is best.

- Consider purchasing a "noisemaker" to block out background noise. It plays soothing sounds of "white noise" or raindrops, ocean waves, etc.

- Limit naps to 10 or 15 minutes during the day. Short naps can be beneficial.

- Listen to tapes of relaxing music or soothing natural sounds if you have trouble falling asleep.

- Jot down problems and set aside a time the next day to focus on them.

- Eliminate intrusive sound and light from your bedroom so you won't be awakened accidentally.

- Sleep in a cool, well-ventilated room (ideal temperature 64° to 66° F)

- Limit caffeine use to no more than 3 cups consumed before 10 a.m.

- Do not smoke after 7 p.m. or quit smoking altogether. **Nicotine has the same effect as caffeine on sleep.**

- Use alcohol lightly. Alcohol can fragment sleep, especially the second half of your sleeping period.

- Avoid heavy meals and heavy spices in the evening. If you have regurgitation problems, raising the head of the bed should help.

- Develop a bedtime ritual. Bedtime reading, unrelated to work, may help relax you.

- If you wake in the night, don't try too hard to fall asleep; rather, focus on the pleasant sensations of relaxation.

- Avoid unfamiliar sleep environments.

- Quality of sleep is important. Too much time in bed can decrease the quality of the next night's sleep.

- Limit the bedroom to sleep and relaxation. Don't use it as a work area.

Figure 4–1. Example of patient handout. (Reprinted with permission, Suzanne M.P. Bennett, D.O., P.C.)

Plan Components

Which of the following would be documented in the plan? Circle all that apply.

physical examination findings   information from medical records

patient education   CBC results   r/o ankle fracture

laboratory and x-ray orders   vital signs   recommended over-the-counter medications

follow-up instructions   review of systems   referrals

Number the following sentences in the suggested order they should appear in the plan.

_____ Discussed the DDX with patient.

_____ Bone densometry.

_____ Ibuprofen 200 mg 1 or 2 every 6 hours PRN pain.

_____ Follow-up in 2 weeks.

_____ CT of chest.

_____ Refer to behavioral health clinic for counseling.

_____ Go to the ED PRN vomiting or increased abdominal pain.

_____ Handout on low back exercises given and explained.

_____ ENT consult.

_____ Albuterol inhaler 1–2 puffs every 4–6 hours PRN wheezing.

These abbreviations were introduced in Chapter 4. Beside each, write its meaning.

PA   _____

ED   _____

D/C   _____

RTC   _____

po   _____

ENT   _____

See Appendix B for the answers to these worksheets.

Office Charting

Purpose

Section 2 introduces you to charting in outpatient care settings. When a patient presents to your office for the first time, a chart must be established. Specific information is required for all patient charts. At a minimum, the baseline clinical data should include a patient history, problem sheet, and medication sheet. Office visits may be for problem-specific, health maintenance, disease and condition monitoring, or follow-up purposes and are generally documented in the progress notes or on specific forms. One chapter each is devoted to pediatric and adult health maintenance visits. Because PAs are found in every specialty, the responsibilities of referring and consulting providers are discussed. Specific situations mandate written patient, parental, or legal guardian consent. Minor office procedures (e.g., biopsies) are the most common situations requiring consent in an outpatient setting.

Objectives

- Describe the contents and organization of an office chart.
- Identify pertinent information that should be on the problem list.
- Initiate and maintain a medication record.
- Compare and contrast the differences between a problem-specific and a health maintenance visit.
- Give examples of when follow-up visits are recommended.
- List conditions in which flow sheets might be useful.
- Understand the responsibilities of the referring and the consulting provider.
- Explain when and why written consent forms are required.
- Locate national guidelines and schedules for common immunizations.
- Describe the components of a pediatric and an adult health maintenance visit.

Chapter 5

New Patients

Establishing a New Patient Record

Patients who are new to the practice fill out several forms that provide basic information required for their medical record. Basic information includes name, address, telephone numbers, date of birth, emergency contact person and phone number, and legal guardian if the patient is a minor or under the care of another person. Financial information, including insurance carrier and the responsible party for payment, is necessary for reimbursement purposes. It is important to familiarize yourself with federal, state, and local requirements for medical record contents. It is usually recommended that billing information and any correspondence regarding billing and payment issues be kept in a separate file.

Patients are usually asked to complete a health history form at their first visit to an office, such as those shown in Figure 5–1 (adult) and 5–2 (pediatric). The form will document much of the patient's past medical history, social history, and family history. This document establishes a database for the patient's health history at that time. It should be reviewed with the patient at the first office visit with follow-up of any positive findings. It is a permanent document in the medical record.

If a patient has medical records from a previous provider, they should be reviewed. These records can be invaluable in filling in the details of a past medical condition. They may contain laboratory tests and x-ray and EKG results that you can compare with current studies. Specialist consultations can provide insight into a disease.

A negative response to previous treatment regimens enables you to try another approach.

An office chart should contain the following records:

- Patient demographic information
- Emergency contact names and numbers
- Financial information, including insurance company, if any
- A problem list
- A medical history
- Progress notes, usually arranged chronologically with the most recent date on top
- A medication record listing all maintenance and PRN medications, nonprescription medications, dietary supplements, drug allergies, and reactions to any medications or supplements
- A section in which preventive health or health maintenance items are documented (often part of the problem list)
- An immunization record
- An area for patient messages

In addition, the following items may be found in a chart:

- Test results: laboratory studies, radiograph or other imaging reports
- Reports from specialists the patient has been referred to, also called consultation notes; this may include therapeutic reports (e.g., from physical or occupational therapists, counselors, psychologists, etc.)
- Hospital, ED, and urgent care clinic records
- Consents for minor surgical procedures done in the office
- Records from previous healthcare providers

To be completed by patient

Date: ___/___/__

Name: _____ Age: _____ Date of Birth: __/__/__ ☐ male   ☐ female

Mailing Address: _____

Home Phone: _____ Work Phone: _____ Other phone: _____

Emergency contact name and phone number: _____

Employer's Name & Address: _____

Please list all the people living in your household and their relationship to you.

Name	Age	Relationship

Personal Health History: Do you have, or have you ever had, any of the following?
(Check all boxes that apply.)

☐ Allergies   ☐ Bowel problems ☐ Heart problems   ☐ Nerve problems
☐ Anemia   ☐ Breathing problems ☐ High blood pressure ☐ Seizures
☐ Alcohol/Drug addiction ☐ Cancer (type____) ☐ High cholesterol ☐ Skin problems
☐ Arthritis   ☐ Depression   ☐ Kidney problems   ☐ Stroke
☐ Asthma   ☐ Diabetes   ☐ Liver problems   ☐ Thyroid problems
☐ Back pain   ☐ Eye problems   ☐ Migraine headaches ☐ Ulcers
☐ Blood transfusion ☐ Serious injury (type_____)

Current Medications (please include prescription and over-the-counter medications):

Name of medication	Dose (mg)	Taken how many times a day?

Medication allergies: ☐ None _____

Please list any hospitalizations or surgeries.

Year	Procedure or Reason for Hospitalization	Doctor	Which hospital

Figure 5–1. Adult medical history form.

Family History: (check all that apply)

	Alcoholism	Asthma or allergies	Cancer (type)	Depression	Diabetes	Heart Disease	High blood Pressure	Stroke	Cause of death	Age at death
Father										
Mother										
Siblings										
Grandparents										

Social History:

Marital status: ☐ married ☐ single

Tobacco use: ☐ none ☐ chew tobacco ☐ cigar/pipe ☐ cigarettes ____

packs/day for _____ years   quit date _____

Alcohol use: ☐ none   drinks/week _____ type of drink: _____

☐ other drug use: (type) _____

Exercise: ☐ daily _____ times/week   intensity: ☐ low ☐ medium ☐ high

☐ aerobic   ☐ weight training

Seat Belt use: ☐ yes ☐ no   Helmet or other safety measures: ☐ yes ☐ no

Immunizations/Screening exams (date of most recent):

☐ hepatitis B ____   ☐ Pneumovax ____   ☐ tetanus ____   ☐ flu shot ____

☐ stool for blood ___ ☐ chest x-ray ___   ☐ TB test ___ ☐ colonoscopy ___

Women only:

Pap Smear _____   Any abnormal Pap smears?   ☐ yes ☐ no

Mammogram _____   Any abnormal mammogram?   ☐ yes ☐ no

Do you perform breast self-exams? ☐ yes ☐ no   If yes, how often? _____

Age you started your periods: _____ Are they regular? ☐ yes ☐ no

Number of days: _____

Do you still have periods: ☐ yes ☐ no   Have you ever taken hormone

replacement therapy? ☐ yes ☐ no

Have you had bone density testing? ☐ yes ☐ no   If yes, when and where

was most recent? _____

How many times have you been pregnant? _____

How many children do you have? _____

Number of vaginal deliveries: _____   Number of C-sections: _____

Men only:

Prostate exam: _____ Any abnormal prostate exams? ☐ yes ☐ no

Testicular exam: _____ Do you perform testicular self-exams? ☐ yes ☐ no

Figure 5–1. Adult medical history form.

To be completed by parent or guardian	Today's Date: ___/___/___

Child's Name: _____ Date of Birth: ___/___/___ ☐ male ☐ female
Mother's Name: _____ Father's Name: _____
Address: _____
Home Phone: _____ Mother's Work Phone: _____ Father's Work Phone: _____
Sibling's names and ages _____
Person completing form/relationship: _____

Birth and Development History:

Mother's age at time of delivery: _____ Type of delivery: ☐ vaginal ☐ Cesarean
Birth weight: _____
Problems during pregnancy: _____ Obstetrician: _____
Feeding: ☐ Breast ☐ Bottle Type of formula: _____ Vitamins: ☐ yes ☐ no

Medical History: (Check if the child has ever had any of the following)

☐ Allergies   ☐ Bladder infection   ☐ Eye problems   ☐ Feeding problems
☐ Anemia   ☐ Breathing problems ☐ Hearing problems   ☐ Skin problems
☐ Asthma   ☐ Bowel problems   ☐ Kidney problems   ☐ Sleep problems
☐ Bedwetting   ☐ Easy bruising/   ☐ Liver problems   ☐ Seizures
                    bleeding
☐ Serious injury (type_____)

Current Medications (please include prescription and over-the-counter medications):

Name of medication	Dose (mg)	Taken how many times a day?

Medication allergies: ☐ None _____

Please list any hospitalizations (other than delivery) or surgeries.

Year	Procedure or Reason for Hospitalization	Doctor	Which hospital

Social History:

Parents' marital status: ☐ married ☐ single ☐ separated ☐ divorced
Any smokers in the house? ☐ yes ☐ no
If divorced or separated, who has legal custody? _____
Car Seat/Seat Belt use: ☐ yes ☐ no   Helmet or other safety measures:
☐ yes ☐ no
Smoke detector in the house? ☐ yes ☐ no   Do you have a pool? ☐ yes ☐ no
If yes, is it fenced? ☐ yes ☐ no

Immunizations (list dates and any severe reactions):

DTP/Td ____ ____ ____ ____ ____ Oral polio ____ ____ ____ ____
MMR ____ ____   HIB-c ____ ____ ____ ____   varicella _____
Cocci (skin test) _____ TB skin test ___

Figure 5–2. Pediatric medical history form.

Problem List

The problem list provides a brief summary of the patient's health status. It is usually one of the first documents you see when you open the chart, enabling you to quickly peruse the list of active and inactive medical conditions and past surgeries. It is important to maintain this list by entering pertinent data as soon as possible. For example, once you receive a bone density report confirming that the patient has osteoporosis or osteopenia, the information should be added to the problem list along with the date. After receiving a discharge summary from the hospital, any newly diagnosed conditions and surgeries should be added to the list. Figure 5–3 illustrates a problem list form. Many healthcare facilities have a standard or customized problem list form that includes the information they deem necessary.

Application Exercise 5.1

Refer to the case study on Mr. Jensen, Chapter 3, Example 3–2. Use these data to complete the problem list shown in Figure 5–3.

APPLICATION EXERCISE 5–1 ANSWERS

Compare your problem list to that in Figure 5–4.

Medication Record

In keeping with the concept of having important patient data available "at a glance" (e.g., the problem list), the medication record provides a summary of the patient's medications. Prescription medications that the patient takes on an ongoing basis and PRN medications should be grouped together by type, when possible. For example, you would list all cardiovascular medications together, all pulmonary medicines together, etc. It is also important to list over-the-counter (OTC) products the patient takes. Many people self-medicate with "natural" or herbal drugs, vitamins, minerals, and other dietary supplements; these should be listed as well.

The medication record should be updated at every office visit to reflect any changes in dosages, directions, or additions or discontinuation of medications. An area to annotate when a

prescription was written, the quantity prescribed, and number of refills is often included. A sample medication record is shown in Figure 5–5.

MEDICOLEGAL ALERT!

Leaving the office with a new prescription is the outcome of many office visits. While the medication record is helpful as a quick reminder of what medications a patient is taking, you should never assume that it is a complete and accurate record. Patients will often start taking medications or may discontinue medications and forget to tell you. It is your responsibility as the provider to determine what medications the patient is taking at every visit and before writing any prescriptions. To meet the standard of care, before prescribing any new medications, you should always ask about current medication usage, including nonprescription medications and dietary supplements, to screen for possible drug-drug interactions. You should explain the expected benefit of taking the medication, educate the patient about potential side effects, and provide any special instructions (such as take with food), and each of these actions should be documented in the plan.

Other data that should be on the medication record include patient's name, date of birth, drug allergies, insurance plan (to alert you to specific drug formularies), and a pharmacy number where the patient regularly fills his or her prescriptions. The date a medication was started indicates how long the patient has been taking a particular medication. When a drug is discontinued, the date and reason why should be documented. This information on the medication record prevents you from having to read through the chart to determine why a medication was stopped. The medication may not have been effective, or the patient may have experienced side effects or developed an allergic reaction. Any drug allergies should be documented, along with the specific reaction, such as rash, hives, itching, difficulty breathing, anaphylactic shock, etc.

Application Exercise 5.2

Using the blank form in Figure 5–5, complete a medication record for Mr. Jensen, based on the information from Chapter 3.

PATIENT: **TEL:**   **SUZANNE BENNETT D.O.**

ICD-9	DATE	CURRENT MAJOR/CHRONIC PROBLEMS	DATE	DX	TREATMENT

DATE	INACTIVE MAJOR PROBLEMS (INCLUDING MAJOR SURGERY)	DATE	DX	TREATMENT

PAP/PELVIC									
BREAST EXAM									
MAMMOGRAM									
GUAIAC									
FLEX/SIG									
COLON									
FLU									
PNEUMO									
TETANUS									
CHOLESTEROL									

Figure 5–3. A blank problem list example. (Reprinted with permission, Suzanne M.P. Bennett, D.O., P.C.)

PATIENT: *JENSEN, William*   TEL: *SCOTT VERNON, MD*

ICD-9	DATE	CURRENT MAJOR/CHRONIC PROBLEMS	DATE	DX	TREATMENT
401.1	*1996*	*HYPERTENSION*	*2/1/04*	*FATIGUE*	*✓ LABS*
272.0	*2001*	*HYPERCHOLESTEROL EMIA*			

DATE	INACTIVE MAJOR PROBLEMS (INCLUDING MAJOR SURGERY)				
1995	*Ⓛ inguinal hernia repair*				
1987	*Torn Ⓡ rotator cuff repair*				

PAP/PELVIC									
BREAST EXAM									
MAMMOGRAM									
GUAIAC									
FLEX/SIG									
COLON									
FLU	*10/2003*								
PNEUMO	*2002*								
TETANUS	*2002*								
CHOLESTEROL	*2002–185*								

Figure 5–4. Problem list example for Mr. Jensen. (Reprinted with permission, Suzanne M.P. Bennett, D.O., P.C.)

Medication Record

LAST NAME	FIRST NAME		M.I.	PHARMACY #		
D.O.B.	HOME #			WORK #		
ALLERGIES:						
Ins. Plan:						

Medication, Dosage, Amount	Date	Date	Date	Date	Date	Date	Date	Date
	Dr./Ref	Dr./Ref	Dr./Ref	Dr./Ref	Dr./Ref	Dr./Ref	Dr./Ref	Dr./Ref

All discontinued medications must be highlighted and remaining blank spaces must be crossed out. Reason for discontinuance of medication must be documented on this record.

Figure 5–5. Medication record.

APPLICATION EXERCISE 5–2 ANSWERS ⎯⎯⎯⎯⎯

Compare your medication record with Figure 5–6.

To reinforce documentation for the new patient and reinforce abbreviations used in this chapter, complete Worksheet 5.1 and 5.2.

Chapter Summary

- New patients are often asked to complete a health history form on their first visit to a practice.

- The chart should be organized in a consistent manner, allowing personnel to quickly find the necessary information.

- The provider should review the medical history form with the patient and follow up on any positive findings in the patient's history.

- The problem list provides a quick summary of the patient's health status.

- The medication record provides a summary of the patient's medications and should be updated at every visit.

- Remember, if it is not documented, it was not done!

Medication Record

Medication, Dosage, Amount	Date	Date	Date	Date	Date	Date	Date	Date
	Dr./Ref	Dr./Ref	Dr./Ref	Dr./Ref	Dr./Ref	Dr./Ref	Dr./Ref	Dr./Ref
Cardizem 120mg	5/17 #30							
SR ÷ po daily	5 RF							
Mevacor 20 mg	5/17 #30							
÷ po daily	5 RF							
Centrum Silver multi-vitamin ÷ po daily								
acetaminophen PRN								
Maalox 2 Tbsp po PRN								

Patient header:

LAST NAME	FIRST NAME	M.I.	PHARMACY #
Jensen	William		555- 0123

D.O.B. xx/xx/xx	HOME # 555- 8760	WORK # Retired

ALLERGIES: Sulfa

Ins. Plan: Medicare

All discontinued medications must be highlighted and remaining blank spaces must be crossed out. Reason for discontinuance of medication must be documented on this record.

Figure 5–6. Completed medication record for Mr. Jensen.

Read the following statements. Place a T for true or an F for false in the space provided on the left next to each statement.

1. ___ Drugs taken on a PRN or "as needed" basis do not need to be listed on the medication record.

2. ___ Progress notes are filed with the first office visit note on top.

3. ___ Correspondence from a physical therapist is filed in the progress notes section of the chart.

4. ___ The medical history form can be discarded once a complete history has been documented in the progress notes.

5. ___ When old records are reviewed, pertinent past medical history should be listed on the problem list.

6. ___ Telephone messages from a patient or family member do not need to be filed in the chart.

7. ___ Drug allergies and the patient's reaction to any medications or supplements should be listed on the medication record.

8. ___ Nonprescription medications do not need to be listed on the medication record.

9. ___ Calcium citrate 600 mg two tabs daily should be recorded on the medication record.

10. ___ Results of a bone density scan should be filed under laboratory tests.

These abbreviations were introduced in Chapter 5. Beside each, write its meaning.

DTP _____

Pap _____

Hib _____

MMR _____

OTC _____

TB _____

Td _____

HS or hs _____

See Appendix B for the answer to these worksheets

Chapter 6

The Office Visit

atiens schedule office visits for a variety of reasons. There may be a specific problem the patient is concerned about, or the visit may be for monitoring an ongoing problem or chronic condition. For clarity and consistency, we will use the term "problem-focused" to refer to a visit for a specific problem and the term "periodic monitoring" for visits that primarily deal with monitoring a chronic condition. Visits may also be scheduled for specific procedures, such as removing skin tags or treating verrucae. The patient may schedule an appointment for a "complete physical," often referred to as health maintenance visits. These types of visits will be discussed in Chapter 7 (pediatric visits) and Chapter 8 (adult visits).

Problem-Focused Visits

A change in the patient's health status usually prompts the patient, or a family member, to call for an appointment. Such changes could include onset of new symptoms, an injury, or concerns and questions about general or specific health issues. When an established patient presents with one of these situations, the SOAP format is frequently used to document this visit. Subjective information for a problem-focused visit should identify the chief complaint and history of present illness. The past medical history, family history, and social history may be pertinent, depending on the chief complaint. The objective information is usually limited to physical examination of the system that parallels with the chief complaint. For instance, the examination of a patient who presents with a sore throat would focus on the HEENT system but would not likely include the abdomen, extremi-

ties, back, or a neurological examination. The assessment and plan would be documented, as discussed in Chapters 3 and 4. Instead of using the SOAP format, some providers may create their own forms for problem-specific visits, such as the one shown in Figure 6–1 that combines text and checklists. Example 6–1 shows a SOAP note for Ms. Naegler, who presented with the specific problem of bilateral heel pain.

EXAMPLE 6–1

PROBLEM-FOCUSED VISIT

S: Ms. Naegler, a 38-year-old female, complains of bilateral heel pain for the past year. She describes a "burning" pain and difficulty walking upon rising in the morning. An achy to sharp pain also occurs with walking, especially on hard surfaces. Pain scale rating: 7/10 in a.m.; 4/10 with walking. There has been no relief with ibuprofen 200 mg two tablets three times a day. Her shoe wear consists of 1-inch heels for work, "flip-flops," and "cheap" tennis shoes. She denies knowledge of any precipitating factors. PMH: Negative for DM. FH: mother has Type 2 DM, controlled with oral agents. SH: quit smoking 2 years ago; 20 pack-year history. Walks a half mile daily with her dog. ROS: negative for fevers, rashes, or injury.

O: WDWN female in NAD.

Ht (Height): 66" Wt (Weight): 170; T 98.2, P 72, R 16, BP 128/66

Lungs: clear to auscultation (CTA).

Heart: regular rate and rhythm (RRR) without murmur or gallop.

Feet: point tenderness to palpation of the anterior calcaneus bilaterally. Rest of foot is nontender. No discoloration; normal temperature; neurovascular system (NVS) intact. Mild pes planus noted bilaterally.

(Continued)

Name _____   Date _____ Time _____

Age _____ Wt _____ Temp _____ P _____ R _____ BP _____ HT _____ Pulse OX _____ LMP _____

Medications ☐ reviewed, no change _____

Allergies _____

CC _____   Time _____

S _____

_____

_____

_____

_____

_____

_____

ROS	NL										
GEN	☐	☐	weakness	☐	fatigue	☐	fever	☐	wt loss/gain	☐	sweats/chills
HEENT	☐	☐	vision loss	☐	eye pain	☐	eye d/c	☐	hearing loss		
		☐	ear pain	☐	sore throat	☐	congestion	☐	runny nose	☐	sinus pressure
RESP	☐	☐	SOB	☐	cough	☐	sputum	☐	hemoptysis	☐	wheezing
BREAST	☐	☐	pain	☐	discharge	☐	mass				
CV	☐	☐	chest pain	☐	PND	☐	orthopnea	☐	palpitations	☐	diaphoresis
GI	☐	☐	abd pain	☐	reflux	☐	N/V	☐	constipation	☐	hematochezia
		☐	melena	☐	diarrhea	☐	dysphagia	☐	heartburn		
EXT	☐	☐	arthralgia	☐	myalgias	☐	back pain	☐	extremity pain	☐	pedal edema
NEURO	☐	☐	HA	☐	numb/ting	☐	weakness	☐	dizzy/vertigo	☐	gait prob
GU	☐	☐	dysuria	☐	frequency	☐	urgency	☐	hematuria	☐	vag bleeding/dc
SKIN	☐	☐	rash	☐	lesion	☐	itch				
PSYCH	☐	☐	depression	☐	anxiety	☐	insomnia				

PMH	☐ rev, no chng	☐ Negative	☐ Angina	☐ Arthritis	☐ Asthma	☐ Back Pain
	☐ Bipolar	☐ CA _____	☐ CHF	☐ COPD	☐ CVA	☐ Depression
	☐ DM 1 2	☐ Diverticulitis/osis	☐ Ectopic preg	☐ GI Bleed	☐ HTN	☐ Hepatitis
	☐ Hyperlipids	☐ MI	☐ Migraines	☐ Ovarian Cyst	☐ Pancreatitis	☐ Pneumonia
	☐ PUD	☐ Pul Emb	☐ PVD	☐ Renal	☐ Seizures	☐ Thyroid
	☐ TIA	☐ Urolithiasis	☐ Other _____			
PSH	☐ rev, no chng	☐ Negative	☐ Chole	☐ Appi	☐ T & A	☐ TAH ___ SO
SOC	☐ rev, no chng	☐ Negative	☐ Alcohol	☐ Drug Abuse	☐ Smkr _____	☐ PPD ____ yrs
FMH	☐ rev, no chng	☐ Negative	☐ Cancer	☐ Diabetes	☐ HTN	☐ Stroke
	☐ MI	☐ Hyperlipids				

A/P _____

_____

_____

_____

_____

_____

_____

_____

_____

Figure 6–1. Sample problem-specific visit form. (Reprinted with permission, Suzanne M.P. Bennett, D.O., P.C.)

Name _____   Date _____

Accompanied by:

Physical Exam

GEN	☐ Wd/Wn/NAD	☐ Awake	☐ Alert
	☐ Oriented	☐ Conversive	☐ Pleasant

BABY	☐ Well Hydrated	☐ Playful
	☐ Fontanelles soft	☐ Sucks well
	☐ Normal Cry	☐ Normal tone

SKIN	☐ Warm/dry/pink	☐ No induration
	☐ No rash	☐ No erythema

HEAD	☐ Sinuses non-tender	☐ Atraumatic

FACE	☐ Temp art non-tender

EYES	☐ PERRL	☐ Conj benign	☐ Non-icteric
	☐ EOMI	☐ Fundi benign	☐ lids wnl.

EARS	Canal	☐ no erythema	☐ no drainage
	TM's	☐ Not red	☐ Not retracted ☐ No perf.

NOSE	☐ No deformities	☐ Not congested
	☐ Pink mucosa	

ORAL	☐ Mucous mem. wnl	☐ No lesions
	☐ lips/teeth/gums wnl.	☐ Moist

Throat	☐ No erythema	☐ No exudates	
	TONSILS	☐ No erythema	☐ No swelling
		☐ No exudates	☐ No abscess

NECK	☐ Supple	☐ Non-tender	☐ Full ROM
	☐ NO stiffness	☐ No nodes	☐ No JVD
	☐ No bruit	☐ No thyroidomegaly	

HEART	☐ Reg rate/rhythm	☐ No murmurs/gallops/rubs
	☐ NO heaves or thrills	☐ PMI wnl

RESP	☐ Breathing	☐ non-labored
	☐ CTA	☐ Chest wall w/o deformity

CHEST	☐ Chest wall non-tender

BREAST	☐ No mass	☐ no nipple d/c	☐ no erythema
	☐ no dimpling	☐ no retraction	☐ symmetrical

ABD	☐ Soft	☐ Non-tender	☐ BS wnl
	☐ No HSM	☐ No rebound	☐ No guarding
	☐ No mass	☐ pos fem pulse	☐ No pulsatile mass

EXTR	☐ Full ROM	☐ No deformity	☐ Non-tender
	☐ No edema	☐ Pulses wnl	☐ Homan sign neg
	☐ No calf tenderness	☐ No clubbing/cyanosis	

BACK	☐ Full ROM	☐ Sensation Feet/legs nl
	☐ Non-tender	☐ SLR neg. bilateral

G/U	☐ No hernia	☐ Penis w/o lesions	
	☐ Testicles w/o tend/mass/swelling		
	☐ Pap done	☐ No CMT	☐ No cervical d/c
	☐ Uterus/adnexa w/o mass/non-tender		

RECTAL	☐ no mass/tend	☐ Prostate wnl
	☐ Stool OB neg	

NEURO	☐ Normal speech	☐ CN 2-12 wnl.
	☐ Reflexes 2+ bilat	☐ Strength 5/5 bilat.
	☐ Sens wnl = bilat.	☐ No nystagmus
	☐ Finger to nose wnl	☐ Heel-shin wnl
	☐ Dicks/Halpike wnl	☐ Babinski down

PSYCH	☐ A&O×3	☐ Memory wnl.
	☐ Mood/Affect wnl.	☐ Judgment/Insight wnl.

Physical Exam (positive findings)/Procedures:

   ☐   >50% time spent counseling patient

Orders	**Labs**	**RAD**
☐ EKG	☐ Fasting	☐ X-Ray
☐ Peak Flow	☐ CBC	☐ U/S
☐ Pulse ox	☐ BMP	☐ CT
☐ Glucose	☐ CMP	☐ MRI
☐ Urine preg	☐ TSH	☐ Mammo
☐ Rapid strep	☐ Lipid Prof	☐ Other
☐ Urine dip	☐ UA C/S	
☐ Spirometry	☐ PSA	
☐ Tympanogram	☐ Other	

Vaccines _____

Referrals _____

Follow Up ___ dys weeks months prn

   ☐ Or if condition persists or worsens

Visit Time _____ minutes

Provider _____ Time _____

   Charge NP 1 2 3 4 5   EP 1 2 3 4 5

Figure 6–1. Sample problem-specific visit form. (Reprinted with permission, Suzanne M.P. Bennett, D.O., P.C.)

![bar]

EXAMPLE 6–1 *(Continued)*

Chart review: had normal CMP, CBC, thyroid-stimulating hormone (TSH), and lipid panel 6 months ago.
A: Heel pain, bilaterally
P: Bilateral heel x-rays. Vioxx 50 mg one po qd pc, PRN pain. #30 tabs, one refill. Report any epigastric or abdominal pain, black bowel movements, or severe heartburn. Handout on heel pain given and explained to patient, including heel stretches and common causes. Avoid walking on hard surfaces. Discontinue (D/C) flip-flops. Recommend she buy a good pair of walking shoes with arch supports. May try heel cushions in shoes. Follow up in 6 weeks.

Follow-Up Visits

Follow-up (F/U) visits provide an opportunity to see how the patient responded to treatment and to discuss whether additional therapy or another course of action is needed. In the example above, Ms. Naegler was asked to follow up in 6 weeks to determine whether she responded to the treatment regimen prescribed. If a patient has been referred to a specialist, the physician assistant (PA) may have them follow up after that consultation visit to discuss any recommended tests or medications. Often, patients are asked to follow up after completing a course of therapy or a trial of medication to see whether their symptoms have resolved or improved.

Patients are often instructed to follow up with their primary care physician after they have been evaluated in an ED or urgent care clinic or after a hospitalization or surgery. To provide continuity of care, medical records from these visits should be available for you to review. Pertinent diagnostic test results should be documented in the objective portion of the note. An example of a follow-up visit for Ms. Naegler is shown in Example 6–2

EXAMPLE 6–2

MS. NAEGLER'S FOLLOW-UP VISIT

S. Ms. Naegler returns for a follow-up on her bilateral heel pain. Overall, she reports approximately 75% improvement. The Vioxx relieves most of her pain. She

has not worn flip-flops since her last visit 6 weeks ago. She has purchased a pair of Rockport walking shoes and has been using OTC heel cushions in her work shoes. She performs her heel stretches every night.
O: NAD. Wt: 165 T 97.8, P 70, R 20, BP 110/62
Lungs: CTA. Heart: RRR without murmur or gallop.
Feet: less tenderness to palpation over the anterior calcaneus. Otherwise, exam unchanged.
Bilateral heel x-rays: small bone spurs @ anterior calcaneus bilaterally.
A: 1) Heel spurs 2) Heel pain: improved.
P: Continue same regimen. Call for Vioxx refills PRN. Ms. Naegler informed that treatment of bone spurs is usually conservative. Other options include orthotics, local cortisone injections, and rarely, surgery, if all medical management fails. F/U if symptoms do not improve over the next 8 to 12 weeks or as needed.

Periodic Monitoring Visits

Many medical conditions should be monitored regularly. The frequency depends upon how stable or unstable each patient's condition is. Complications of the condition and potential side effects of certain medication or therapeutic treatment modalities influence the type and frequency of monitoring. Healthcare organizations, such as the cancer societies, diabetes societies, and federal government agencies, periodically publish their recommendations for monitoring. We do not attempt to dictate the details of these visits, merely to make you aware of them. It is your responsibility to determine the national, regional, and local medical community's standard of care guidelines.

For certain conditions, such as diabetes, or when a patient takes certain medications, such as warfarin, a flow sheet may be helpful. Flow sheets are an excellent "at a glance" method of reviewing the patient's blood sugar levels or laboratory results obtained when a patient takes certain medications (Figure 6–2). Some medications that may be tracked using a flow sheet include warfarin or anticoagulant therapy, insulin, and Depo Provera injections. Conditions in which flow sheets may be helpful in monitoring the patient's response to therapy include diabetes and hyperlipidemia.

COUMADIN / ANTICOAGULANT FLOW SHEET

Name _____   Date Coumadin Started _____

Phone _____   Diagnosis _____

DATE	Coumadin Dose (mg)	INR	Protime	Coumadin New Dose	When to Recheck	Remarks

Figure 6–2. Coumadin/anticoagulant flow sheet. (Reprinted with permission, Suzanne M.P. Bennett, D.O., P.C.)

In the assessment part of the SOAP note, you can describe the status of the chronic condition, such as "Type 2 diabetes improved," or "uncontrolled," or "stable."

MEDICOLEGAL ALERT!

Checklists must be used appropriately. Do not check something unless you asked about that system or performed that function. Do not commit fraud.

Application Exercise 6.1

Using the problem-specific form provided in Figure 6–1, document Ms. Naegler's initial visit.

APPLICATION EXERCISE 6.1 ANSWERS

Compare your completed form to that shown in Figure 6.3.

Patient's Noncompliance with Treatment

Occasionally, despite efforts to treat patients, they may not follow the treatment plan that you recommend. A patient may deliberately choose not to follow the treatment plan or may not be able to for some reason. If a patient did not follow the treatment plan, you should attempt to determine why; document this conversation with the patient. The patient may not be able to afford the medication you prescribed, or the treatment plan may conflict with the patient's cultural or spiritual beliefs. Your responsibility as a provider is to educate the patient about the benefits and risks of the treatment plan and potential consequences of not following treatment recommendations. It is not the provider's responsibility to force patients to do something they do not want to do, even if you do not understand the reason or agree with the reason. Your responsibility lies in providing competent advice and in documenting discussions with the patient regarding noncompliance.

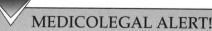

MEDICOLEGAL ALERT!

It is crucial to document noncompliance in the patient's medical record. If you do not, and the patient has a poor outcome, the patient or a family member may sue you. The patient or family may claim that you did not appropriately care for the patient. You must document that you counseled the patient about her health condition and warned her of potential morbidity and mortality. Whenever possible, use direct quotes from the patient when documenting noncompliance and refrain from making any judgmental statements about the patient.

Consultations and Referrals

When a second opinion is sought from another healthcare provider, it is called a consultation. For example, you have a patient with a constellation of symptoms and abnormal tests. The differential diagnoses have been narrowed down to three possible diagnoses. A consultation is requested, with the purpose of narrowing the differential diagnoses even further or arriving at the definitive diagnosis. The consultant's role is to recommend further diagnostic testing or make a diagnosis and recommend a plan of care. Typically, the patient will visit the consultant one or two times.

Transferring responsibility to another healthcare provider for the treatment of a specific problem is called a referral. For example, a 13-year-old boy presents with a fracture of the distal tibia that involves the epiphysis. He is referred to an orthopedic specialist for fracture care. The specialist chooses and carries out the treatment modalities. Upon recovery, the patient may be released from the specialist's care, or periodic follow-up visits may be recommended to monitor his progress and response to treatment.

The terms consultation and referral are sometimes used interchangeably, even though there is a distinct difference. To clarify the role of each provider, reference may be made to the referring physician and the consulting physician. It is the referring physician's responsibility to specify the reason for the referral and the action desired so that the consulting physician knows whether it is for an opinion only or also involves management. Pertinent information must be trans-

Name _Melinda Naegler_ _____   Date _9-14-03_   Time _9:40 a.m._

Age _38_ Wt _170_ Temp _98.2_ P _72_ R _16_ BP _128/66_ HT _66"_ Pulse _OX_ _99%_ LMP _9-3-03_

Medications ☐   reviewed, no change _Ibuprofen 200mg 2 TID prn_ _____

Allergies _____

CC _c/o bilateral heel pain × 1yr_ _____   Time _____

S _c/o "burning pain & difficulty walking upon rising in A.M._

 c/o achy to sharp pain c̄ walking, especially on hard surfaces.

 Pain scale rating: 7/10 in A.M. 4/10 c̄ walking.

 o relief c̄ ibuprofen

 Shoewear: 1 inch heels for work, "flip-flops" & "Cheap" Tennis shoes.

 Denies any precipating factors, Denies injury.

 QD 1/2 mile walks c̄ small dog.

ROS	NL					
GEN	☒	☐ weakness	☐ fatigue	☐ fever(−)	☐ wt loss/gain	☐ sweats/chills
HEENT	☐	☐ vision loss	☐ eye pain	☐ eye d/c	☐ hearing loss	
		☐ ear pain	☐ sore throat	☐ congestion	☐ runny nose	☐ sinus pressure
RESP	☐	☐ SOB	☐ cough	☐ sputum	☐ hemoptysis	☐ wheezing
BREAST	☐	☐ pain	☐ discharge	☐ mass		
CV	☐	☐ chest pain	☐ PND	☐ orthopnea	☐ palpitations	☐ diaphoresis
GI	☐	☐ abd pain	☐ reflux	☐ N/V	☐ constipation	☐ hematochezia
		☐ melena	☐ diarrhea	☐ dysphagia	☐ heartburn	
EXT	☐	☐ arthralgia	☐ myalgias	☐ back pain	☒ extremity pain	☐ pedal edema
NEURO	☐	☐ HA	☐ numb/ting	☐ weakness	☐ dizzy/vertigo	☐ gait prob
GU	☐	☐ dysuria	☐ frequency	☐ urgency	☐ hematuria	☐ vag bleeding/dc
SKIN	☒	☐ rash(−)	☐ lesion	☐ itch		
PSYCH	☐	☐ depression	☐ anxiety	☐ insomnia		

PMH	☐ rev, no chng	☒ Negative	☐ Angina	☐ Arthritis	☐ Asthma	☐ Back Pain
	☐ Bipolar	☐ CA ___	☐ CHF	☐ COPD	☐ CVA	☐ Depression
	☐ DM 1 2(−)	☐ Diverticulitis/osis	☐ Ectopic preg	☐ GI Bleed	☐ HTN	☐ Hepatitis
	☐ Hyperlipids	☐ MI	☐ Migraines	☐ Ovarian Cyst	☐ Pancreatitis	☐ Pneumonia
	☐ PUD	☐ Pul Emb	☐ PVD	☐ Renal	☐ Seizures	☐ Thyroid
	☐ TIA	☐ Urolithiasis	☐ Other ___			
PSH	☐ rev, no chng	☒ Negative	☐ Chole	☐ Appi	☐ T & A	☐ TAH ___ _SO_
SOC	☐ rev, no chng	☐ Negative	☐ Alcohol	☐ Drug Abuse	☐ Smkr _T_	☐ PPD _20_ yrs _Quit 2001_
FMH	☐ rev, no chng	☐ Negative	☐ Cancer	☒ Diabetes	☐ HTN	☐ Stroke
	☐ MI	☐ Hyperlipids		_mom-type 2_		

A/P _HEEL PAIN, Bilat_   _√ bilat heel x-rays_ _____

 Rx Vioxx 50mg 1 po QD pc PRN pain #30 tabs 1 Refill

 Report any epigastric or abd pain, black BM, severe heartburn.

 Handout on heel pain Given & explained to pt, including heel

 stretches & common causes. Avoid walking on hard surfaces.

 D/C flip flops. Recommend pt buy a good pair of walking shoes,

 c̄ arch supports. May try heel cushions in shoes F/U 6 wks

Figure 6–3. Completed problem-specific visit form for Ms. Naegler. (Reprinted with permission, Suzanne M.P. Bennett, D.O., P.C.)

Name _MELINDA NAEGLER_   Date _9-14-03_

Accompanied by: ø

Physical Exam

GEN	☑ Wd/Wn/NAD	☐ Awake	☐ Alert		
	☑ Oriented	☐ Conversive	☐ Pleasant		
BABY	☐ Well Hydrated	☐ Playful			
	☐ Fontanelles soft	☐ Sucks well			
	☐ Normal Cry	☐ Normal tone			
SKIN	☑ Warm/dry/pink	☐ No induration			
	☑ No rash	☐ No erythema			
HEAD	☐ Sinuses non-tender	☐ Atraumatic			
FACE	☐ Temp art non-tender				
EYES	☐ PERRL	☐ Conj benign	☐ Non-icteric		
	☐ EOMI	☐ Fundi benign	☐ lids wnl.		
EARS	Canal	☐ no erythema	☐ no drainage		
	TM's	☐ Not red	☐ Not retracted ☐ No perf.		
NOSE	☐ No deformities	☐ Not congested			
	☐ Pink mucosa				
ORAL	☐ Mucous mem. wnl	☐ No lesions			
	☐ lips/teeth/gums wnl. ☐ Moist				
Throat	☐ No erythema	☐ No exudates			
	TONSILS	☐ No erythema	☐ No swelling		
		☐ No exudates	☐ No abscess		
NECK	☐ Supple	☐ Non-tender	☐ Full ROM		
	☐ NO stiffness	☐ No nodes	☐ No JVD		
	☐ No bruit	☐ No thyroidomegaly			
HEART	☑ Reg rate/rhythm	☑ No murmurs/gallops/rubs			
	☑ NO heaves or thrills	☐ PMI wnl			

RESP	☐ Breathing	☑ non-labored		
	☑ CTA	☐ Chest wall w/o deformity		
CHEST	☐ Chest wall non-tender			
BREAST	☐ No mass	☐ no nipple d/c	☐ no erythema
	☐ no dimpling	☐ no retraction	☐ symmetrical
ABD	☐ Soft	☐ Non-tender	☐ BS wnl
	☐ No HSM	☐ No rebound	☐ No guarding
	☐ No mass	☐ pos fem pulse	☐ No pulsatile mass
EXTR	☑ Full ROM	☑ No deformity	☐ Non-tender
	☑ No edema	☑ Pulses wnl	☐ Homan sign neg
	☑ No calf tenderness	☑ No clubbing/cyanosis	
BACK	☐ Full ROM	☐ Sensation Feet/legs nl	
	☐ Non-tender	☐ SLR neg. bilateral	
G/U	☐ No hernia	☐ Penis w/o lesions	
	☐ Testicles w/o tend/mass/swelling		
	☐ Pap done	☐ No CMT	☐ No cervical d/c
	☐ Uterus/adnexa w/o mass/non-tender		
RECTAL	☐ no mass/tend	☐ Prostate wnl	
	☐ Stool OB neg		
NEURO	☑ Normal speech	☐ CN 2-12 wnl.	
	☐ Reflexes 2+ bilat	☐ Strength 5/5 bilat.	
	☐ Sens wnl = bilat.	☐ No nystagmus	
	☐ Finger to nose wnl	☐ Heel-shin wnl	
	☐ Dicks/Halpike wnl	☐ Babinski down	
PSYCH	☑ A&O×3	☐ Memory wnl.	
	☑ Mood/Affect wnl.	☐ Judgment/Insight wnl.	

Physical Exam (positive findings)/Procedures:

☐ >50% time spent counseling patient

Chart review: Normal CMP, CBC. TSH & lipids 3/03.

FEET: Point tenderness to palpation of anterior calcaneus bilat. Rest of foot non tender. ø discoloration. Normal temperature of feet. Mild pes planus bilat.

Orders	Labs	RAD
☐ EKG	☐ Fasting	☑ X-Ray _B heels_
☐ Peak Flow	☐ CBC	☐ U/S
☐ Pulse ox	☐ BMP	☐ CT
☐ Glucose	☐ CMP	☐ MRI
☐ Urine preg	☐ TSH	☐ Mammo
☐ Rapid strep	☐ Lipid Prof	☐ Other
☐ Urine dip	☐ UA C/S	
☐ Spirometry	☐ PSA	
☐ Tympanogram	☐ Other	

Vaccines _____

Referrals _____

Follow Up _6_ dys weeks months prn

☐ Or if condition persists or worsens

Visit Time ___15___ minutes

Provider _Lynnette, PAC_ Time _____

Charge NP 1 2 3 4 5   EP 1 2 3 4 5

Figure 6–3. Completed problem-specific visit form for Ms. Naegler. (Reprinted with permission, Suzanne M.P. Bennett, D.O., P.C.)

mitted to consulting physicians for their review when patients present for their appointments. This may consist of a written summary, progress notes, problem list, medication sheet, flow sheets, diagnostic testing, other consultant's notes, and hospital discharge summary. If imaging studies have already been done, the consulting physician may wish to view the actual films, so patients may need to be instructed to obtain those films and take them to the appointment. Duplication of tests should be avoided unless deemed necessary by the consulting physician.

The referring physician maintains responsibility for the health of the patient, even when he or she is under a specialist's care. Consulting physicians are expected to communicate with the referring physician in a timely manner. The initial consultation note typically resembles a complete history and physical, impression or assessment, and recommended plan of care. If the patient is to remain under the consulting physician's care, follow-up notes should be sent apprising the referring physician of the patient's progress.

Consent is required before performing any invasive procedures. According to *Stedman's Medical Dictionary*, 26th edition, "invasive" is defined as "a procedure requiring insertion of an instrument or device into the body through the skin or a body orifice for diagnosis or treatment." Consent may be documented in the SOAP note, or a specific consent form may be used, such as the one shown in Figure 6–4. Certain injections, such as local cortisone injections and immunizations, require consent. Minor office procedures include all types of skin biopsies (shave, punch, excisional), ingrown toenail removals, incision and drainage (I&D) of abscesses, and excision of skin lesions (e.g., sebaceous cysts). If there is a question about whether a consent form is needed, try applying the definition of "invasive." If there is still doubt, obtain the consent.

A written consent form must be completed and signed by the patient before performing invasive procedure. The consent form has many functions. It explains what the procedure is, who will perform it, and why it is being done; lists the possible complications of performing the procedure; and contains the patient's signature confirming their consent. Most consent forms have space for a witness to sign as well. If the patient disagrees with a clause in the consent form, he or she may cross it out and initial it. The provider must then decide whether the disagreement is acceptable and whether they will proceed with or cancel the procedure.

To further reinforce concepts related to documentation of office visits please complete Worksheets 6.1 and 6.2 at the end of this chapter.

Chapter Summary

- Most office visits are problem-specific.
- Problem-specific visits are usually for illness, injury, a new symptom or problem, or concerns and questions.
- Components of the problem-specific progress note include chief complaint, HPI, pertinent PMH (including FH and SH), a focused physical examination, an assessment, and a plan.
- Having the patient return for a follow-up visit enables you to assess the patient's response to treatment and provides an opportunity for further patient education.
- Patients are often advised to follow up with their primary care practitioner after hospitalization and after a visit to the emergency department, urgent care clinic, therapist, specialist, or other healthcare provider.
- Periodic monitoring visits are important in chronic diseases. The frequency depends on the stability of the patient's condition.
- Flow sheets allow you to quickly review the course of a patient's condition. They aid in revealing trends that may not be noticed by reading through the progress notes.
- A progress note may be documented on a plain sheet of paper or on a preprinted form.
- Referring and consulting providers have specific responsibilities to facilitate positive patient outcomes.
- Informed consent allows patients to make educated decisions about their health care.
- Invasive procedures require written consent from the patient, parent, or legal guardian.
- Remember, if it is not documented, it was not done!

Bennett Family Medicine

Name _____   Date _____

I hereby give my informed consent for the following surgical procedure:

Shave Bx   Punch Bx   Skin tag removal   Wart destruction

Curettage/ dessication   Excision   Liquid Nitrogen destruction of precancers

Other: _____

This procedure has been fully explained to me by Dr. Bennett/staff, including the reasons for this procedure, other options available and inherent risks of the procedure and anesthesia, if required, including complications or side effects that might result. I understand the more common risks of any surgical procedure include rare reaction to local anesthesia, pain or discomfort, bleeding, infection, scar, and even possibly the need for further surgery. I understand that if I experience any problems subsequent to this procedure that I am to notify Dr. Bennett immediately so that they may optimize my care and minimize any potential short term serious or long term adverse effect or outcome. I have been given the opportunity to ask questions of Dr. Bennett/staff and have had all questions or concerns answered to my satisfaction prior to the procedure.

Signed _____

Printed Name _____

Witness _____

Figure 6–4. Consent form. (Reprinted with permission, Suzanne M.P. Bennett, D.O., P.C.)

1. List three general reasons why a patient would schedule a problem-specific office visit.

_____

_____

_____

2. Mrs. Gonzalez, an established patient, presents to your office with a chief complaint of "Right elbow swelling × 2 days."

   Which of the following statements do NOT belong in this problem-specific progress note? (Circle all that apply.)

   Patient hit her elbow on the corner of a coffee table

   Mother alive and well, 74 years old, HTN × 25 years

   Hospitalized age 22 for pneumonia

   Bursitis, right elbow, secondary to trauma

   Patient denies history of IV drug abuse

3. List six components of a problem-specific progress note. Example: chief complaint.

   _____

   _____

   _____

   _____

   _____

   _____

4. Give four reasons why a patient would be advised to schedule a follow-up visit.

   _____

   _____

   _____

   _____

5. Explain the purpose of flow sheets.

   _____

   _____

6. Name three conditions under which flow sheets might be a useful tool.

_____

_____

_____

7. Evaluate the following statements. Place a T for true or an F for false in the space provided.

___ The frequency of periodic monitoring visits depends on the stability of the patient's condition.

___ Use of a checklist to document an office visit is considered fraudulent.

___ A referral is used if you want a second opinion from another healthcare provider.

___ The referring provider is responsible for transmitting pertinent patient information to the consulting provider.

___ When patients undergo a minor procedure, they must sign a consent form.

These abbreviations were introduced in Chapter 6. Beside each, write its meaning.

CTA _____

RRR _____

IV _____

NVS _____

TSH _____

F/U _____

qd _____

CVA _____

LDL _____

HDL _____

I&D _____

See Appendix B for the answers to these worksheets.

Chapter 7

Pediatric Health Maintenance Visits

$\mathcal{P}$ediatric health maintenance visits, or well child visits, are often enjoyable for the provider and may provide an opportunity for you to interact with a patient who is not "ill." In obtaining the subjective information, you will often have to rely on parents or caregivers of the patient to provide the medical history. Because children at certain ages are unable to voice their problems or concerns, you may have to rely more heavily on the objective data you obtain during a visit than you would for a visit by patients who are able to vocalize their needs. Observing the child and interactions between the child and others becomes an important part of the objective portion of the pediatric health maintenance visit.

Age is an important consideration when conducting and documenting well-child visits. Age is documented in months when the child is 24 months or younger and in years and months for children older than 24 months (e.g., "17 months," and "3 years, 8 months"). We consider anyone under the age of 18 to be a pediatric patient. During the first 2 years of life, periodic well-child visits are generally recommended at the ages of newborn and 1, 2, 4, 6, 9–12, and 15–18 months. Once a child reaches the age of 24 months, well child visits are recommended at least once during the age ranges of 2–3, 4–5, 6–9, 10–13, and 14–18 years. Girls should be seen annually once they reach menarche, and boys and girls should be seen annually once they are sexually active.

The well child visit may be documented in the SOAP format presented in Section I or on preprinted forms. Such forms make documentation easy and efficient with fill-in-the-blank and checklist features while ensuring thoroughness, proper billing, and reduced liability exposure. The American Academy of Pediatrics has developed a set of Pediatric Visit Documentation Forms for well child visits from the initial visit at 2 weeks of age up to the 2-year well child visit. The forms may be viewed and ordered from the organization's website at www.aap.org. Health history forms such as the one shown in Figure 5–2 can also be used.

Components of Pediatric Health Maintenance Visits

The components of well child visits generally follow the format of the complete history and physical examination (Table 1–1 and Figure 2–1, respectively), with minor variations related to age. Other components of pediatric health maintenance visits include:

- Growth screening
- Developmental screening
- Appropriate laboratory screening tests
- Assessing immunization status and administering as appropriate
- Anticipatory guidance, counseling, and education
- Risk-factor identification

Growth Screening

Growth and development are important parameters that should be assessed routinely during well child visits. Growth generally refers to the increase in size of the body as a whole or its separate parts. Growth charts are used to assess and compare a child's growth with a nationally representative reference population and are available for boys, birth to 36 months; girls, birth to 36 months; boys 2 to 20 years; and girls, 2 to 20 years. Growth charts provide an overview of the normal growth trajectory of children, thus alerting the provider to what is atypical or disturbed. Standardized growth charts are available from the Centers for Disease Control and Prevention (CDC) and can be viewed at and downloaded from the organization's Website at www.cdc.gov.growthcharts. The measurements typically recorded during the first 2 years of life are length (or height), weight, and head circumference. After the age of 2 years, head circumference may not be measured at every visit if the child's development has been consistent.

A sample growth chart for plotting length and weight for age is shown in Figure 7–1. To plot the length, find the age across the top of the length graph and then find the length in inches along the left axis. Follow each line to the intersecting point and mark. To plot the weight, find the child's age across the bottom of the weight graph and the weight in pounds along the right axis. Follow each line to the intersecting point and mark. You will notice lines curving across the chart with small numbers corresponding to each line at the right side of the chart. These numbers refer to percentiles. Percentile is the most commonly used clinical indicator to assess the size and growth patterns of individual children in the United States. Percentiles rank the position of an individual by indicating what percentage of the reference population the individual would equal or exceed. For example, on the weight-for-age growth charts, a 5-year-old girl whose weight is at the 25th percentile weighs the same or more than 25 percent of the reference population of 5-year-old girls and weighs less than 75 percent of 5-year-old girls.

Weight is an important measurement to document over a person's life. Weight is one parameter used to calculate the body mass index (BMI). BMI is calculated from weight and height measurements (wt/ht^2) and is used to judge whether individuals' weight is appropriate for their height. BMI should be used beginning at 2 years of age, when an accurate stature can be obtained, to screen for overweight children. BMI calculators are readily available on-line at various Websites. The CDC, together with the National Center for Health Statistics, developed a graph for plotting BMI percentiles. It is shown in Figure 7–2 and is available at www.cdc.gov/growthcharts.

Application Exercise 7.1

On the sample growth chart shown in Figure 7–1, plot the length and weight for Kevin, a 21-month-old boy. His length is 33 inches, and his weight is 29 pounds. Determine Kevin's percentile for length and weight.

APPLICATION EXERCISE 7.1 ANSWER

Compare your marks on the graph with those shown in Figure 7–3. Kevin's weight is in the 50th percentile, and his length is in the 75th percentile.

Developmental Screening

Development refers to changes in function, including gross- and fine-motor, language, and psychological functions. Developmental screening includes subjective information from parents and caregivers and objective information observed by the clinician. If a child fails to meet developmental milestones at the appropriate age or if there is any suspicion of developmental delay, formal developmental testing may be warranted. There are numerous developmental tests that can be used for this purpose, such as the Denver Developmental Screening Test-II (DDST-II). There are specific scoring instructions for the DDST-II, and it is usually administered only by specially trained persons and at specific testing agencies. You should consult a pediatric textbook for more information on the DDST-II.

Laboratory Screening Tests

Metabolic screening: State law may mandate various metabolic screening for conditions

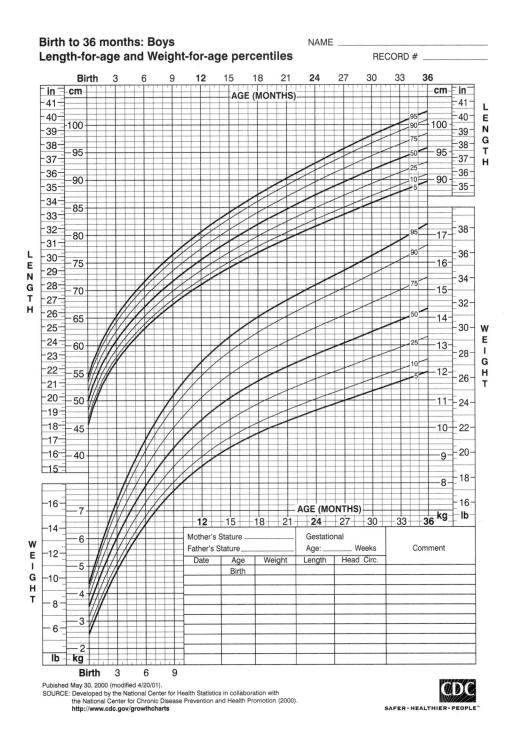

Figure 7–1. A sample growth chart. (Developed by the National Center for Health Statistics in Collaboration with the National Center for Chronic Disease Prevention and Health Promotion [2000] and modified 4/20/01.)

2 to 20 years: Girls
Body mass index-for-age percentiles

NAME _____

RECORD # _____

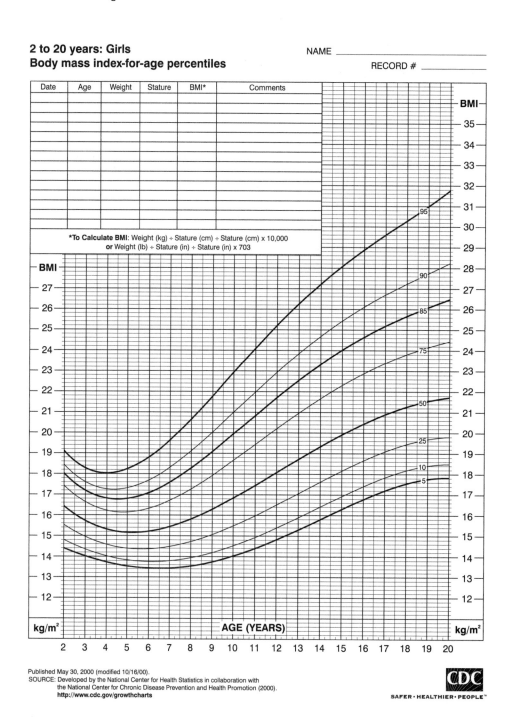

Published May 30, 2000 (modified 10/16/00).
SOURCE: Developed by the National Center for Health Statistics in collaboration with
    the National Center for Chronic Disease Prevention and Health Promotion (2000).
    http://www.cdc.gov/growthcharts

CDC
SAFER · HEALTHIER · PEOPLE™

Figure 7–2. Body mass index graph. (Developed by the National Center for Health Statistics in Collaboration with the National Center for Chronic Disease Prevention and Health Promotion [2000] and modified (10/16/00.)

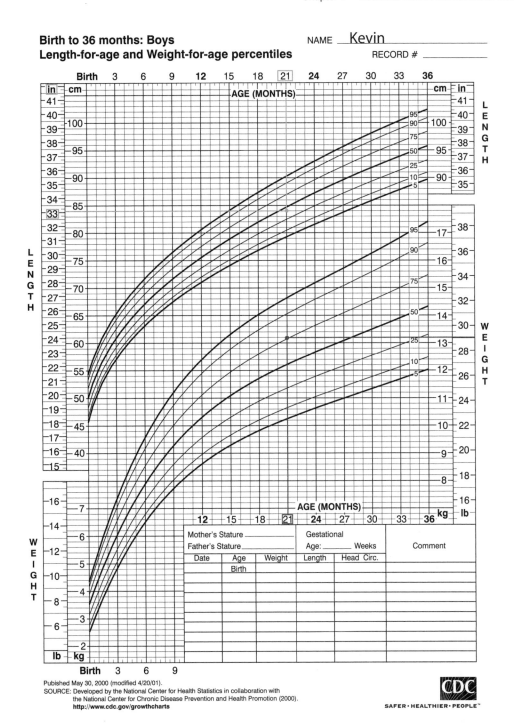

Birth to 36 months: Boys
Length-for-age and Weight-for-age percentiles

NAME ___Kevin___

RECORD # _____

Figure 7–3. A sample growth chart showing Kevin's weight and length. (Developed by the National Center for Health Statistics in Collaboration with the National Center for Chronic Disease Prevention and Health Promotion [2000] and modified 4/20/01.)

such as thyroid disorders, hemoglobinopathies, phenylketonuria (PKU), and galactosemia. Many of these tests are administered at the hospital before the infant's discharge. States may require certain screenings to be performed more than once. We recommend that you consult your state public health department to determine your state's required screenings and schedules.

Anemia screening: Recommended between 9 and 12 months, between 2 and 5 years, and annually after menarche for girls.

Urinalysis: Dipstick screening for leukocytes is recommended annually for any sexually active male or female.

Lead screening: The CDC recommends routine screening between the ages of 9 and 12 months and again at 24 months, but public health authorities in each state are responsible for setting state and local policy on childhood lead screening. A screening questionnaire of three questions may also be used to determine whether lead screening is needed. Children whose parents respond "yes" or "not sure" to any of these three risk-assessment questions should be considered for screening:

1. Does your child live in or regularly visit a house or child care facility built before 1950?

2. Does your child live in or regularly visit a house or child care facility built before 1978 that is being or has recently been renovated or remodeled?

3. Does your child have a sibling or playmate who has or had lead poisoning?

Assessing Immunization Status

Every pediatric visit, whether for well child care or sick child care, is an opportunity to assess the child's immunization history and determine whether immunizations need to be administered. The CDC and the National Immunization Program publish recommendations for childhood and adolescent immunizations. They also publish a catch-up schedule for children who were not immunized at the recommended ages. The recommendations are usually updated annually, and we encourage you to visit the CDC's Website at www.cdc.gov to obtain the most current schedule.

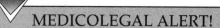

MEDICOLEGAL ALERT!

Some parents or guardians may not want their child to receive immunizations. If a parent/guardian refuses immunizations, you should ask why they are refusing. The parents may have misinformation about the risks of immunizations, they may not understand the reason for immunizations, or they may refuse immunizations because of cultural or religious beliefs. It is important to provide education to the parents about the benefits and risks of immunizations, but ultimately, the parents have the right to refuse immunizations. Any attempts you make at educating the parents on the benefits and risks of immunizations should be documented, along with any written material or other resources you may have given the parents.

Anticipatory Guidance

Anticipatory guidance refers to specific topics that should be discussed with parents and caregivers of pediatric patients at age-appropriate levels. As children grow and develop, we anticipate that they will be involved in certain activities. For instance, many children learn to ride bicycles around 4 to 5 years of age. Anticipating that this may occur should prompt you to educate parents and caregivers that they should talk to the child about bicycle safety, wearing a helmet, wearing reflective clothing, etc. Table 7–1 presents topics that should be addressed with parents and caregivers based on the age of the child. Be sure to document which topics you discussed with the parent/caregiver.

Risk-Factor Identification

If a patient has a family history of certain high-risk diseases, such as tuberculosis and cholesterol, early screening may be recommended. You can consult professional organizations or the CDC for the most current screening guidelines. Screening for sexually transmitted diseases should be performed at least annually for all sexually active patients, including pelvic examination for female patients.

Table 7–1 Age-Specific Anticipatory Guidance*

Age at Visit	Topics to Discuss
Newborn ___ days to 2 weeks	
	Good parenting practices; postpartum adjustment; infant care/sleep positioning; injury prevention; closeness with the baby, individuality of infants, breast/bottle feeding; signs of illness
1 month	Injury prevention; sleep practices; sleep positioning; bladder and bowel habits; nutrition; infant development; when to call the doctor; infant care; plans for next visit
2 months	Injury prevention; nutrition; sleep positioning/practices; fever education; family relationships; other child care providers; talk to baby; pacifiers, bottle tooth decay
4 months	Injury prevention; choking, aspiration; teething; solid foods; sleep positioning; thumb sucking; baby-proof home; appropriate child care providers
6 months	Injury prevention; cup, finger foods; no bottle in bed; pool and tub safety; teething; poisons—ipecac; nutrition; sleep positioning
9–12 months	Baby-proof home and pool; shoes – protection, not support; talk to child; self-feeding; sleep; discipline; praise; dental hygiene
15–18 months	Safety; tantrums; eating; discipline/limits; sleeping; snacks; dental hygiene; no bottles; sibling interaction; read to child; toilet training; aspiration
2–3 years	Decreased appetite, brushing teeth; toilet training; read to child; independence/dependence; car, home, and swimming pool safety; preschool; control of TV viewing
4–5 years	Preschool and school readiness (attention span, easy separation from parents); seat belts; street safety; should know full name, address, and phone number; household chores; no playing with matches; sexual curiosity
6–9 years	Water, seat belts, skate board, and bicycle safety; dental hygiene; peer relations; nutrition; limit setting; regular physical activity; parental role model; communication
10–14 years	Safety issues; nutrition; dental hygiene; peer pressure; smoking, alcohol, and drugs; puberty; safe sex/contraception/STD prevention; communication
15–18 years	Safety issues; dental hygiene; smoking, alcohol, and drugs; safe sex/contraception/STD prevention; communication, dating, peer pressure, motor vehicle safety; sports safety; staying in school

*Adapted from Early Periodic Screening Diagnosis and Treatment (EPSDT) program guidelines. The EPSDT is a national Medicaid program. More information is available at http://www.hcfa.gov/medicaid/epsdthm.htm

Age-Specific Well Child Visits

The content of the physical examination of pediatric patients includes each of the systems shown in Figure 2–1. You are encouraged to follow the "head to toe" order when conducting a physical examination, but exceptions are made for pediatric patients. If possible, you should auscultate the lungs, heart, and abdomen when the child is quiet and not crying. Some components of the examination are likely to elicit crying, such as examining the ears and the oropharynx and conducting parts of the musculoskeletal examination. Regardless of the order in which the examination is performed, you should always document in the order shown in Figure 2–1.

Many excellent references are available that teach physical examination techniques. It is beyond the scope of this book to present the

entire physical examination for all the age-specific well child visits. Once a child reaches school age, the physical examination is essentially the same as the adult physical examination. Table 7–2 presents a summary of physical examination components that should be documented specifically when performing infant and toddler examinations. Table 7–3 shows neurological reflexes that should be tested and documented during infancy. If you detect any abnormalities on physical examination, be sure that your assessment and plan address what additional testing, if any, is indicated and what follow-up will be needed. Worksheet 7.1 will help assess your understanding of pediatric health maintenance visits. Worksheet 7.2 will give you more exposure to the medical abbreviations used in this chapter. Both worksheets can be found at the end of this chapter.

Table 7–2 Documentation of Important Components of Age-Specific Physical Examinations

System Examination Component	Age	Comments
Skin		
Color for jaundice, cyanosis, other discoloration	All ages; most critical in neonate	Jaundice that appears within the first 24 hours of birth is likely to be pathologic jaundice due to hemolytic disease of newborn; jaundice that persists beyond 2–3 weeks should raise suspicions of biliary obstruction or liver disease; important to document presence or absence of Mongolian spot, because it may be misdiagnosed as ecchymosis, raising concern of intentional injury
Rash or lesions	All ages	Many benign skin lesions and rashes common in childhood
HEENT		
Head	Birth until sutures and fontanelles closed	Anterior fontanelle at birth measures 4–6 cm in diameter, closes between 4 and 26 months of age; posterior measures 1–2 cm at birth, usually closes by 2 months
Eyes	Birth to 24 months	
Red reflex		Absence may indicate congenital glaucoma, cataract, retinal detachment, or retinoblastoma
Strabismus		If present after 10 days of age, may indicate poor vision or central nervous system disease
Mouth		
Teeth	First eruption, then throughout life	First eruption around 6 months, then usually a tooth each month until 2 years, 2 months
Tonsils	All ages	May be enlarged in healthy child; peak growth of tonsillar tissue between 8 and 16 years
Palate	Most critical in infancy	Document whether any cleft or bifid uvula
Neck		
Lymph nodes	All ages	May not be palpable until toddler
Nuchal rigidity	All ages	Not a reliable sign of meningeal irritation until after age of 2 years
Respiratory		
Lung sounds	Every visit	Look for a cause of any abnormal breath sounds
Cardiovascular		
Heart rate, rhythm, and sounds	Every visit	Document character of any murmur present and include in assessment and plan; Still's murmur common in preschool- and school-age children, usually benign
Gastrointestinal		
Umbilical cord	Birth until healed	Document that parent/caregiver was educated on cord care
Bowel sounds	Every visit	Absence of bowel sounds is always abnormal; look for cause
Rectum	Birth	Assess and document patency

Table 7–2 Documentation of Important Components of Age-Specific Physical Examinations

System Examination Component	Age	Comments
Male genitourinary		
Testes	Most critical at birth	Both testes should be descended; if cannot palpate both, consultation is warranted
Scrotum	Most critical at birth	Inspect for masses; if present, document whether transparent on transillumination; hydroceles common in newborns
Penis, including foreskin	All ages	Nonretractable at birth, but must visualize the urinary meatus and document presence or absence of hypospadias; document sexual maturity using Tanner's stages*
Female genitourinary		
Breasts	All ages	In newborn, may express white liquid for up to 2 weeks; document breast development
External genitalia	All ages	Often a milky-white or blood-tinged vaginal discharge in first few weeks; inspect hymen; document external genital development using Tanner's stages*
Musculoskeletal		
Clavicle	Birth	Fracture may occur during delivery
Spine	Birth through adolescence	Assess for spina bifida at birth, and screen for scoliosis until adolescence
Hips	Birth through 6 months	Document findings of Barlow and Ortolani tests; if there is congenital hip dysplasia, the best outcome is when treatment is initiated in the first 6 weeks of life
Neurological		
Cranial nerves	Birth to 24 months, then annually if normal	Consult physical examination reference for strategies to assess cranial nerves in newborns, infants, and young children
Reflexes		Many reflexes present at birth will disappear in infancy; see Table 7–3 for reflexes that should be tested in infancy

*Refer to a physical diagnosis reference for explanation and more information

Pediatric Sports Participation Physical

Many pediatric patients will want to participate in sports activities and usually will need medical clearance to be able to do so. The preparticipation physical examination is often the only time a healthy adolescent will see a medical professional, so it is important to include some age-appropriate screening questions and anticipatory guidance. All components of an age-specific physical examination should be completed, with particular emphasis on the respiratory, cardiac, and musculoskeletal systems. The recommended musculoskeletal examination is provided in Table 7–4.

◾ Chapter Summary

- The focus of pediatric health maintenance, also referred to as well child examinations, is on the assessment and documentation of growth and development.

- Important measures during the first 2 years of life include head circumference, length (or height), and weight. From ages 2 to 20, BMI should be determined and graphed. Charts for both may be obtained at the CDC website (www.cdc.gov/growthcharts).

Table 7–3 Neurological Reflexes that Should be Tested During Infancy*

Reflex	Ages	Comments
Palmar grasp	Birth to 3–4 months	Persistence beyond 4 months suggests cerebral dysfunction
Plantar grasp	Birth to 6–8 months	Persistence beyond 8 months suggests cerebral dysfunction
Moro (startle reflex)	Birth to 4–6 months	Persistence beyond 4 months suggests neurological disease; persistence beyond 6 months is strongly suggestive of disease; asymmetric response suggests fracture of clavicle, humerus, or brachial plexus injury
Asymmetric tonic neck	Birth to 2 months	Persistence beyond 2 months suggests neurological disease
Rooting	Birth to 3–4 months	Absence of rooting indicates severe generalized or central nervous system disease
Placing and stepping	4 days after birth, variable age to disappear	Absence of placing may indicate paralysis; babies born by breech delivery may not have placing reflex
Parachute	Develops around 4–6 months and does not disappear	Delay in appearance may predict future delays in voluntary motor development
Trunk incurvation (Galant's reflex)	Birth to 2 months	Absence suggests a transverse spinal cord lesion or injury

*Refer to a physical examination reference for a full description of each reflex and maneuver to elicit.

Table 7–4 Musculoskeletal Portion of Sports Preparticipation Physical Examination

Examination Component and Maneuver	Assessment
Neck: move neck in all directions	Range of motion
Shoulders – shrug against resistance	Test strength of shoulder, neck, and trapezius muscles
Arms – hold out to side and apply pressure	Strength of deltoid muscle
Arms – hold out to side, bend 90° at elbows, raise and lower arms	External rotation and stability of glenohumeral joint
Arms – hold out straight then bend and straighten elbow	Range of motion of elbow
Arms – hold down, bend 90° at elbows, pronate and supinate forearm	Range of motion of elbows and wrists, muscle strength of forearms and wrists
Hand – make a fist, clench and then spread fingers	Range of motion of fingers, strength and stability of joints and muscles
Squat and duck walk	Hip, knee, and ankle range of motion; joint strength and stability
Stand straight with arms to side, back to examiner	Symmetry, leg-length discrepancy
Bend forward from waist with knees straight	Scoliosis of spine
Stand and raise up on toes and walk on heels	Ankle joint strength and stability and calf muscle strength

- The components of a pediatric health maintenance visit include a comprehensive history, physical examination, assessment and plan, growth and development screening, appropriate laboratory screening tests, assessment of immunization status and immunization administration as needed, anticipatory guidance, and risk-factor identification and screening.
- The CDC has established guidelines for immunizations, and the most current immunization recommendations may be accessed at the organization's website, at www.cdc.gov.

- Age-specific guidelines are available for the history, physical examination, and anticipatory guidance.
- The preparticipation sports physical examination may be the only time a healthy child or adolescent seeks medical attention, so age-appropriate history, physical examination, and anticipatory guidance should be part of the sports physical
- Remember, if it is not documented, it was not done!

1. List five components of pediatric health maintenance visits.

_____

_____

_____

_____

_____

2. List three growth parameters that should be measured and documented from birth to 24 months of age.

_____

_____

_____

3. Sexually active pediatric patients should be screened for which of the following? Circle the correct answers

anemia   galactosemia   urinalysis

lead   STDs

4. Name three widely used resources available from the CDC.

_____

_____

_____

5. Which statement is true?

a. The pediatric physical examination may be completed in any order and documented in any order.

b. The pediatric physical examination may be performed in any order but should be documented in head-to-toe order.

These abbreviations were introduced in Chapter 7. Beside each, write its meaning.

EPSDT _____

BMI _____

CDC _____

DDST-II _____

PKU _____

See Appendix B for the answers to these worksheets.

Chapter 8

Adult Health
Maintenance Visits

Kristin Foulke, MPH, PA-C, contributing author

$\mathcal{T}$here are many similarities between pediatric health maintenance visits and adult health maintenance visits. Although the focus of the pediatric health maintenance visit is on growth and development, the focus of the adult visit is on health promotion and disease prevention. Health promotion is general and broad in scope and applies to the adult population at large. Disease prevention is narrower in focus and is individualized according to a person's age, race, gender, medical history, social history, and personal and family risk factors.

There are many reasons to promote health and prevent disease. It is easier to prevent a disease than treat it. The cost for disease management creates a tremendous economic burden for government payers and private insurance carriers as well as society in general. In addition to the economic cost of disease, there is tremendous influence on individuals' and their families' quality of life. Current screening recommendations are focused on preventing, diagnosing, and treating the diseases that occur most frequently and that have the highest morbidity and mortality rates.

Many federal and state agencies and specialty organizations, such as the American Heart Association and the American Cancer Society, publish guidelines for disease prevention. Although many recommendations are the same, variations in frequency of screening exist. It is beyond the scope of this book to include all the recommendations that have been published; instead, the most generally accepted guidelines are summarized.

■ Components of an Adult Health Maintenance Visit

The components of adult health maintenance visits generally follow the format of the complete history (Table 1–1) and physical examination (Figure 2–1). Components of adult health maintenance visits include:

- Risk-factor identification based on personal and family history
- Appropriate laboratory and diagnostic screening tests
- Gender-specific screening
- Assessment of immunization status and administering as appropriate
- Patient education and counseling

Preprinted forms, such as the one shown in Figure 5–1, may be used to collect much of the patient's history, including personal and family medical history. Patients who are new to a practice are often asked to complete a health history questionnaire at their first visit. If such a form is used, it is important that you take the time to review the form thoroughly with the patient and follow up on any existing problems.

Risk-Factor Identification Based on Personal History

Inquiry about and documentation of certain items in the history will help identify personal risk factors. Documenting detailed personal history information will remind you of topics that should be addressed when providing patient education and counseling later in the visit. Inquiring about some of these areas could appear judgmental. It is a good idea to let patients know that you ask all patients these questions. Approaching these matters in a non-judgmental, professional, matter-of-fact manner should enhance patient disclosure of sensitive information.

Height and Weight

Body mass index (BMI) should be calculated and plotted on a BMI chart such as the one shown in Figure 7–2. Increasing morbidity is associated with increasing BMI. At the prevention visit, it is important to explore why the patient is obese and encourage a healthy lifestyle through weight management, nutrition, and exercise.

Exercise

This concerns type (e.g., walking, weight lifting, aerobics), frequency, and duration (e.g., 30 minutes every other day). Lack of exercise or a sedentary lifestyle is a risk factor for certain conditions.

Diet

This involves usual daily food intake, fad diets, dietary supplements, and food allergies, (such as lactose intolerance). Analyze for nutritional excesses and deficiencies, such as high fat, high sugar, low fruit and vegetable intake or inadequacies in a vegetarian diet. Document the quantity of caffeine consumed per day in standard units of measure, such as how many cups of coffee or tea, number of colas, and amount of caffeine-containing foods.

Alcohol Use

Document type of alcohol, amount, and frequency. If the patient discloses any alcohol consumption, it is customary to screen for alcoholism using the CAGE questionnaire:

C Have you ever felt the need to **C**ut down on drinking?

A Have people **A**nnoyed you by criticizing your drinking?

G Have you ever felt **G**uilty about drinking?

E Have you ever taken a drink first thing in the morning (**E**ye-opener) to steady your nerves or get rid of a hangover?

Alcoholism is suggested by two or more "yes" answers, necessitating further inquiry or referral. Any effect on home or work life strongly suggests alcoholism.

Tobacco Use

Document type used (cigarettes, chewing, pipe, cigar), amount used per day, and how long the patient has been using tobacco. Documentation of the brand of cigarettes indicates the amount of nicotine intake. For example, light cigarettes contain less nicotine than unfiltered cigarettes. Cigarette use is usually reported as a "pack-year history." This figure is determined by multiplying the number of packs smoked per day by the total number of years smoked. If the patient quit smoking, note the year quit and the pack-year history. If a patient is currently smoking, it is important to counsel the patient on the health risks associated with tobacco use.

Application Exercise 8.1

Calculate the pack-year history for a patient who has smoked for 20 years and smokes 2 packs per day (PPD). _____

APPLICATION EXERCISE 8.1 ANSWER

The patient has a 40 pack-year history. (20 years x 2 PPD = 40 pack-year history)

Other Substance Abuse

Document type of substance used, frequency of use, and route of administration. Specifically inquire about intravenous (IV) drug abuse. Ask about substances that have a high potential for abuse, such as hypnotics, anxiolytics, prescription or over-the-counter diet pills, narcotic analgesics, and synthetic drugs (Ecstasy, methamphetamine).

Sexual History

Document the age at onset of sexual activity; number and gender of partners; history of sexually transmitted diseases (STDs), such as gonorrhea, chlamydia, herpetic infections, human immunodeficiency virus (HIV), syphilis, pelvic inflammatory disease, and hepatitis; and at-risk behaviors, such as promiscuity and lack of condom use.

Safety

Use of seat belts, motorcycle or bicycle helmets, and other safety devices should be documented. You should also inquire whether there is a smoke detector in the home and safe storage and removal of firearms. Other safety measures that should be documented are use of sunscreen and avoiding the use of alcohol while driving.

Domestic Violence

Patients rarely volunteer that they are victims of domestic violence, but they will often answer truthfully if you bring up the subject. It is important to ask about domestic violence in a nonjudgmental and caring manner. Instead of asking, "Are you being abused?" you could ask, "Do you feel safe at home?" Any positive response should be documented and addressed with appropriate patient education and referral information.

Dental Health

In conjunction with a complete oral physical examination, it is important to encourage regular visits to a dentist and inquire about flossing, brushing, and fluoride toothpaste use.

Psychiatric History

Include dates, diagnoses, hospitalizations, and treatment for any mental or emotional disorder and any suicidal thoughts or attempts.

Personality traits, such as anger or a history of violence, should be documented.

Blood Transfusions

Determine dates of and reasons for the transfusions. Ask about HIV and hepatitis status. Include any history of needle sticks in healthcare personnel, along with testing, treatment, and prophylactic measures taken.

Occupational History

Inquire about exposure to chemicals and environmental conditions, such as noise, that may affect the patient's health.

Risk-Factor Identification Based on Family History

A detailed family history is a key component of a health maintenance visit. Many illnesses are directly linked to a genetic predisposition. It is sometimes tempting to order every test available, but this is not a cost-effective approach nor is it in the best interest of the patient. Focusing specifically on conditions or diseases that are part of your patient's family history is a more reasonable approach. When obtaining the family history, be sensitive to the patient's emotions. Patients might have fears and concerns about conditions or diseases that run in their family. Table 8–1 lists common diseases that have a familial tendency and the preliminary tests that should be used to screen each disease.

Appropriate Laboratory and Diagnostic Screening Tests

Various governmental agencies and specialty societies, such as the American Cancer Society and the American Heart Association, publish recommendations for periodic screening tests. Insurance companies may have their own schedules for screening tests. It is beyond the scope of this book to discuss all the screening tests that could be performed, but general screening recommendations are presented. Many of the recommended screening tests are

Table 8–1 Common Diseases and Recommended Screenings

Family History	Recommended Screening Test
Cancer	
Breast	Clinical breast examination
	Mammogram
Ovarian	Bimanual pelvic examination,no recommended screening test, ultrasound and carcinoembryonic antigen (CEA) if there is clinical suspicion
Prostate	Digital rectal examination
	Prostate specific antigen (PSA)
Colon	Fecal occult blood test (FOBT)
	Sigmoidoscopy or colonoscopy[1]
Heart Disease	
Hypertension	Blood pressure evaluation
Hyperlipidemia	Diet evaluation, Cholesterol panel
Psychiatric Disease	
Depression	Psychiatric history
	Depression screening evaluation
Schizophrenia	Psychiatric history
Suicide	Psychiatric history
	Depression screening evaluation
Alcoholism	CAGE questions
Autoimmune Disease	
Rheumatoid arthritis	History and physical examination
	Rheumatoid factor (RF)
	Sedimentation rate
Systemic lupus erythematosus	Antinuclear antibody (ANA)
	Sedimentation rate
Endocrine Disease	
Diabetes	Fasting blood sugar (FBS)
	Glucose challenge test[2]
	Hemoglobin A_{1c} (HgbA$_{1c}$)[2]
Thyroid Disease	Thyroid-stimulating hormone (TSH) T3[2]
	Free T4[2]

[1]Patients who have a family history of colon cancer should have a colonoscopy rather than a sigmoidoscopy.
[2]If clinically indicated.

appropriate for the general adult population. These are shown in Table 8–2. Other tests are gender-specific and are discussed in the next section. Determining which screening tests to order is based on conditions and diseases that the patient is at risk for as revealed by the medical history.

◼ Gender-Specific Screening

The Female Examination

In addition to the history and physical examination that you will perform for all adult well visits and the screening recommendations outlined in Table 8–2, the female health maintenance visit typically includes additional diagnostic studies. The female health maintenance visit, often referred to as a well woman examination (WWE), includes breast and pelvic examinations. Other screening examinations, such as those shown in Table 8–3, may be clinically indicated.

When performing a clinical breast examination, it is appropriate to educate the patient about how to perform a breast self-examination. Patient education about normal findings at the time of the examination helps the patient become familiar with her body and detect any changes that might occur. Document any patient education in the plan, even if you perform this at the same time you are doing a physical examination. The plan may also include an order for a mammogram if clinically indicated.

Pelvic examinations are performed for screening of STDs and female cancers. A Papanicolaou test will be obtained as part of the pelvic examination for the purpose of screening for cervical cancer. Bimanual pelvic examination will be performed to search for any adnexal masses. It is important to document whether there is any difficulty performing any part of a pelvic examination. Some patient characteristics may lead to a clinically unsatisfactory examination. The patient may be anxious and unable to relax, or the patient may be very obese, and it may be difficult or even impossible to palpate some anatomic structures. For instance, if a patient is morbidly obese and you are unable to palpate the ovaries, you may not be able to detect an ovarian mass. Rather than simply omitting the part of the examination that was difficult or unsatisfactory, you should document the difficulties encountered and describe why the examination was unsatisfactory. If a patient refuses any part of the examination or refuses to have a screening test that is indicated, you should document the patient's refusal in the

Table 8-2 Screening Recommendations

Screening Test	Recommended Ages	
	Male	**Female**
Total cholesterol	35–65 [1]	45–65 [1]
Venereal disease research laboratory (VDRL)	20+[2]	20+ [2]
Flexible sigmoidoscopy	50+ [3]	50+ [3]
Colonoscopy	50+ [3,4]	50+ [3,4]
Digital rectal examination	40+ [5]	40+ [5]
FOBT	40+ [6]	40+ [6]
EKG	40+ [2]	40+ [2]
CXR	20+ [2]	20+ [2]
TSH	20+ [2]	20+ [2]
CBC	20+ [2]	20+ [2]
CMP	20+ [2]	20+ [2]
Fasting blood sugar	20+ [2]	20+ [2]
Urinalysis (UA)	20+ [2]	20+ [2]
Hearing Assessment	20+ [2]	20+ [2]
PPD	20+ [2]	20+ [2]
Glaucoma screening	Refer high-risk patients to eye specialist for screening	Refer high-risk patients to eye specialist for screening

[1]Unless clinically indicated earlier by history.
[2]If clinically indicated.
[3]Fecal occult blood testing should precede the decision to perform a flexible sigmoidoscopy or colonoscopy. Positive fecal occult blood testing would indicate a colonoscopy instead of a flexible sigmoidoscopy. Recommended every 5 years.
[4]Colonoscopy for high-risk individuals as indicated by history, every 10 years.
[5]At the time of the flexible sigmoidoscopy or colonoscopy.
[6]Annually.

Table 8-3 Screening Recommendations for Females

Screening Test	Frequency
Pelvic examination	Performed in conjunction with a Pap test in patients that have a cervix, after age 40 annually.
Papanicolaou (Pap) test	Pap testing recommended every 3 years after two normal annual tests for all women who have been or are sexually active and who have a cervix. If the patient is taking contraceptive medication or hormone replacement therapy, annual Pap tests are performed. No evidence has proven the upper age limit to discontinue Pap testing.
Clinical breast examination	Every 3 years from age 20 to 40 unless clinically indicated.
Mammogram	Annually after age 40 years, sooner if clinically indicated.
Rubella serology or vaccination	Women of child-bearing age
Bone density scan	65 years+; sooner if clinically indicated.

appropriate system (i.e., if the patient refuses the rectal examination, document in the genitourinary system) or in the plan if a recommended test is refused.

THE MALE EXAMINATION

The male health maintenance visit, also called the well male examination, should include a genital examination and inguinal hernia check as well as the general physical examination. For men over the age of 40 years, a prostate and rectal examination should be performed, as indicated in Table 8–4. The stool should be tested for occult blood, which is typically documented in the physical examination section. If the patient refuses to allow any part of the examination, be sure you document appropriately.

Table 8–4 Screening Recommendations for Males

Screening Test	Frequency
Prostate-specific antigen screening	Annually after age 50 years
Prostate examination	Annually after age 50 years
Testicular examination	18+
Hernia examination	18+

MEDICOLEGAL ALERT!

You may read a chart where some part of the examination has been "deferred." There are few occasions where this should occur. It is not appropriate to document "deferred" if you, as the provider, do not want to perform the examination. Likewise, it is not appropriate to document "deferred" if the patient refuses the examination. In some instances, it is medically advisable to defer part of the examination. For instance, if a patient is having acute chest pain and dyspnea, it would be medically acceptable to defer the rectal examination because positioning the patient to perform the examination may exacerbate the patient's condition and cause unneeded distress. If you defer any part of the examination, document the reason why, and do not leave it open to speculation as to why the examination was deferred.

Assessing Immunization Status

Immunization status review is an important component of the adult health maintenance visit. Immunizations are important to prevent disease and should be maintained through adulthood. Many patients are not aware of the need for vaccines unless they are required for certain activities, occupations, or college entrance. If your patient was fully immunized during childhood, immunizations that they are likely to need as adults include diphtheria-tetanus, hepatitis B, influenza, and pneumonia. If your patient was not fully immunized during childhood, a catch-up schedule is available. The Centers for Disease Control and Prevention (CDC) is the best source for up-to-date information on adult immunizations, schedules, and the medical indications for specific immunizations. You may access this information at www.cdc.gov

Patient Education and Counseling

The health maintenance visit is a convenient time to educate and counsel patients. Any patient education or counseling provided should be documented in the plan portion of the SOAP note. It is important to reinforce and praise patients for positive health behaviors and equally important to educate patients about the risks associated with negative health behaviors, such as smoking. Because smoking is likely to continue over time, ongoing education about the risks of smoking and counseling the patient regarding the benefits of not smoking is likely to be a part of every visit. Studies have shown that the healthcare provider's advice can have a strong influence on patient behavior. Patients may not be ready to change their behavior at any particular visit, but they may move closer to making a change when the information is reinforced in multiple visits.

MEDICOLEGAL ALERT!

Documenting that you have counseled the patient on the risks of negative health habits and the management of chronic disease is an important part of medicolegal risk management. Remember, if it is not documented, it has not been done! Providers have been sued for not providing patient education and counseling. One such case involved a physician assistant and a 33-year-old woman. The patient was obese and hypertensive, and she smoked. She had frequent visits to the clinic for various complaints. Routine screening tests revealed marked hypercholesterolemia and an abnormal high-density:low-density lipoprotein (HDL/LDL) ratio. The physician assistant (PA) never counseled the patient regarding her risk for coronary artery disease, and never reviewed the case with the supervising physician. Several years later, the patient presented to an emergency room with crushing chest pain that radiated to her arms and neck. The diagnosis of myocardial infarction was confirmed, but by the time the diagnosis was made, the window of opportunity for thrombolytic therapy had closed. The patient sued the clinic and the PA for malpractice. The PA was found negligent for not educating and counseling the patient about her risk factors for developing heart disease.

A negative health behavior that is a risk factor for a condition should be listed in the assessment portion of the SOAP note, and any patient education or counseling provided should be in the plan portion. For example, if a patient smokes, "tobacco dependence" would be listed as an assessment, and the plan would read "educated patient on health risks of smoking and advised smoking cessation." The patient's response to the counseling should also be documented in the plan. If you advise smoking cessation and the patient says "I'm not ready to quit yet," you should document this response using the patient's exact words. It is a good idea to provide written information to patients. You can develop your own patient education materials or provide materials developed by specialty organizations (such as the American Cancer Society, CDC, American Heart Association). Be sure to document what specific patient education material was provided to the patient and encourage the patient to call you with any questions about the information provided or to discuss them at the patient's next visit.

Worksheet 8.1 will help reinforce the documentation discussed in this chapter, and Worksheet 8.2 will give you more practice with the abbreviations used in this chapter.

Chapter Summary

- Screening for conditions and diseases should be based on the patient's personal and family history.
- Many specialty organizations and payer groups have developed recommendations for screenings. Only a summary of the most common recommendations has been included here.
- Immunization status should be assessed at adult health maintenance visits. The most current recommendations may be accessed at www.cdc.gov
- The assessment portion of the SOAP note should include conditions associated with negative health behaviors.
- Patient education and counseling is an important part of every adult health maintenance visit and should be documented in the Plan portion of the SOAP note.
- Praise the patient for positive health behaviors and offer on-going patient education and counseling related to negative health behaviors.
- Remember, if it is not documented, it was not done!

Section 3

Hospital Charting

Purpose

Section 3 introduces you to charting in an inpatient setting. When a patient is admitted to the hospital, a flurry of paperwork ensues. The admitting physician or designee is required to conduct and document the admission history and physical within 48 hours of admission. During a hospital stay, the medical staff is responsible for seeing patients on a daily basis (rounds) and documenting their response to any treatment being provided. When a patient's condition has improved, the medical staff is responsible for discharging the patient. A specific type of documentation accompanies each of these activities. State and federal regulatory agencies have specific requirements for hospital documentation. These requirements have been incorporated into generally used formats like the ones presented here. Some hospitals have additional requirements or slightly different formats, and the medical records department will be able to furnish you with its required format.

Objectives

- Identify the components of an admission history and physical.
- Use a mnemonic device to write admission orders.
- Identify typical admission orders for medical and surgical admissions.
- Document a hospitalized patient's daily progress using the SOAP format.
- Write orders that reflect changes in a patient's care during a hospital stay.
- Write a discharge summary and corresponding discharge orders.
- Document special activities, such as procedures, patient leaving hospital against medical advice, etc.

Chapter 9

Admitting a Patient to the Hospital

Creating a Record

Some of the records you create related to a patient's hospital admission, such as daily orders and progress notes, will be hand-written. Other records, such as the admission history and physical and the discharge summary, will be dictated. The dictated information will be transcribed, and the transcribed copy will become part of the medical record. It can be intimidating when you first start dictating, but as with most other skills, the more you do it, the easier and less intimidating it becomes. An important truth to keep in mind is that you do not have to get everything perfect the first time. If you make a mistake, you simply rewind and re-record the information. Most institutions have written guidelines for dictation, and often step-by-step instructions are displayed prominently in dictation areas. If you are unable to locate instructions, ask a member of the medical records staff to assist you. Some suggestions for dictating records follow:

- Organize your thoughts and your materials before you begin to dictate. This will help decrease the amount of time you spend going through the chart hunting for specific information.

- Speak slowly and clearly. Try to reduce background noise as much as possible.

- Get in the habit of doing a "sound check" at the beginning of a dictation session. Record a few words, then play back the recording to check for clarity of your speech, volume, background noise, and other factors that will influence the quality of your dictation.

- Always spell out patient's names, even if it is a very common name, such as Mary. It is also a good ideal to spell out the names of any physicians or other healthcare providers who were involved in the patient's care. It is good practice to spell out the names of medications, especially ones that are not used frequently or new medications.

- If you need to look through the chart for information, use the pause feature on the dictation system. Transcriptionists do not want to listen to you thumbing through pages of a chart. It puts unnecessary gaps in the dictation and can be very distracting.

- When you are dictating, do everything possible to avoid having a conversation at the same time. If someone walks up and asks you a question about Mrs. Smith while you are dictating a record on Mrs. Jones, the answer you provide may inadvertently become part of the medical record for Mrs. Jones. Transcriptionists are responsible for typing out information that is heard on the tape; they are not responsible for editing tapes as they transcribe.

- Remember to protect the patient's confidentiality as much as possible. Be aware of who is within hearing range when you are dictating. If others are in the immediate area, especially other patients or family members of patients and there is a chance that they may overhear your dictation, move to a more private area to dictate to avoid violating confidentiality.

The Admission History and Physical

One of the most important documents generated for a patient's hospital stay is the admission history and physical, often referred to as the H&P. Numerous members of the health-care team use information in the H&P as the cornerstone of patient care. The Joint Commission on Accreditation of Healthcare Organizations (JCAHO) requires that an admission H&P contain identification data, the patient's chief complaint, details of the present illness, relevant past medical, social and family histories, an inventory of body systems (review of systems, or ROS), a thorough physical examination, a statement of the conclusions or impressions drawn from the history and physical examination, and a statement of the course of action planned for the patient while in the hospital. An admission H&P may be performed up to 7 days before a planned admission and up to 48 hours after an admission.

The contents of the H&P should seem familiar to you and can be reviewed in Chapter 1 and in Table 1–1. You can review the objective data from the physical examination and laboratory studies in Chapter 2 and in Figure 2–1. In the admission H&P, include the admitting diagnosis and a brief treatment plan that outlines what care the patient will receive during hospitalization. The admitting diagnosis or diagnoses may be listed as presumptive diagnoses. For instance, a patient presenting with chest pain may have a presumptive diagnosis of acute myocardial infarction. It may take additional time and testing to confirm the diagnosis, so in scenarios like this, a presumptive diagnosis is usually more appropriate. A brief outline of the patient's plan of care should be provided. The plan of care is communicated by writing the appropriate admission and daily orders.

Types of Admissions

An admission for treatment of pneumonia or sepsis or other problems treated primarily with medical rather than surgical therapy is considered a medical admission. A hospitalization for an elective or necessary surgical procedure is considered a surgical admission. Much of the paperwork and patient care is the same, but each type of admission has some distinct characteristics. It is helpful to understand the differences between surgical and medical admissions when writing admission orders and documenting the patient's daily progress.

If not before admission, the admission H&P should be completed within 48 hours of admission. In most hospitals, you will complete the H&P and then dictate the information. The admission H&P discussed above is for the patient admitted to the hospital for 24 hours or more. It is common for patients to have surgical procedures as outpatients and never be admitted to the hospital. This is called *same-day surgery* or *outpatient surgery*. In these instances, an abbreviated H&P may be used. Many hospitals and freestanding surgical centers have their own same-day or outpatient surgery H&P form. A sample same-day surgery H&P form is shown in Figure 9–1.

The Admit Note

When records are dictated, there is often a 24- to 48-hour delay between the time of dictation and when the record appears on the chart in its final form. Because of this delay, it is customary to write a brief admit note in the chart. The purpose of the admit note is to summarize the admission H&P and to provide information that will be needed to care for the patient until the dictated records get to the chart. Document that an admission H&P has been performed and dictated, indicating the date and time it was done. This informs other medical staff members that the H&P has been done so that it will not be duplicated. It also serves as documentation that the H&P has been completed in the required time.

The admit note is a permanent part of the medical record. As such, it should be thorough enough to communicate the reason for the patient's hospitalization and should include the presumptive diagnosis and treatment plan, but keep in mind that it is a brief summary of the H&P. An admit note typically contains the patient's identifying information, reason for admission, pertinent past medical history, medications, allergies, pertinent physical examination findings, pertinent laboratory data, admitting diagnosis, and a summary of the treatment plan. It is usually written as a narrative paragraph. Here is one example of an admit note.

Central Medical SurgiCenter

1333 N. 30th St.

Central City, US

Phone: 802-555-4400 Fax: 802-555-4801

Same Day Surgery History and Physical Form

Patient's Name: _____   MR#: _____

DOB: _____   Gender: [ ] male [ ] female

Diagnosis: _____

Surgical Procedure: _____

Surgeon: _____

Anesthesia: [ ] general   [ ] local   [ ] other _____

Pertinent HPI: _____

Medications: _____

Allergies: _____

Chronic Medical Conditions: _____

Pre-Op Labs: (check box for desired tests)

[ ] HGB   [ ] HCT   [ ] CBC   [ ] UA   [ ] EKG

[ ] CXR   [ ] CMP   [ ] glucose   [ ] PT   [ ] INR (International
                                                          Normalized Ratio)

[ ] other: _____

Vital Signs: ___ BP   ___ pulse   ___ resp.   ___ temp

EXAM: [ ] well developed, well nourished [ ] A&O $\times$ 3   [ ] no distress

HEENT: [ ] normal   [ ] abnormal _____

Neck: [ ] normal   [ ] abnormal _____

Lungs: [ ] normal   [ ] abnormal _____

Heart: [ ] normal   [ ] abnormal _____

Abd: [ ] normal   [ ] abnormal _____

Ext: [ ] normal   [ ] abnormal _____

Neuro: [ ] normal   [ ] abnormal _____

Cleared for surgery?   [ ] yes   [ ] no

Consent to read: _____

Consent signed? [ ] yes   [ ] no   NPO?   [ ] yes   [ ] no

Figure 9–1. Sample same-day surgery history and physical form.

EXAMPLE BOX 9-1

Admit note: Ms. Blanchard is a 72-year-old woman who developed symptoms of fever and cough 2 days ago and has had progressive dyspnea. Her past medical history is significant for COPD and hypertension. She takes Accupril 10 mg daily and uses a Combivent inhaler twice daily. On physical examination, she is febrile and dyspneic but not cyanotic. Crackles are heard in the right posterior lung. Heart is tachycardic but regular, with a rate of 112. Chest x-ray reveals a right lower lobe (RLL) infiltrate. Presumptive diagnosis is RLL pneumonia. Ms. Blanchard is admitted to the medical service with IV antibiotic therapy and supportive respiratory care.

For more practice with admit notes, look at the admit note in Worksheet 9.1 at the end of this chapter. Identify the information according to the elements usually included in an admit note, and then check your answers.

Admit Orders

When a patient is admitted to the hospital, the orders written at the time of admission will direct the health-care team in caring for the patient. It is important that the orders be completed in a timely manner and that they be legible, thorough, and unambiguous. Once written, an order is considered to be in effect until an order is written to change or stop the original order, unless a time limit is provided in the original order. An order to record intake and output would be carried out until an order is written to discontinue intake and output. An order for *Ancef 1 g IV q 24 hrs × 3 days* will be given only for 3 days, and it is not necessary to write an order to stop Ancef.

There are several mnemonics that may be used to help you remember what admission orders should be written. One mnemonic is AD CAVA DIMPLS, which stands for **A**dmit, **D**iagnosis, **C**ondition, **A**ctivity, **V**ital signs, **A**llergies, **D**iet, **I**nterventions, **M**edications, **P**rocedures, **L**abs, and **S**pecial instructions. Each component is described in more detail, and an example of each is provided. Figure 9–2 presents the mnemonic in a condensed form.

Admit

Specify the admitting physician and which hospital unit the patient should be admitted to.

Admit to Dr. Johnson to the orthopedic floor or *Admit to Dr. Myers to telemetry unit.*

Diagnosis

State the admitting diagnosis and, in the case of a surgical admission, include the name of the procedure to be performed. When a patient has more than one admitting diagnosis, the problem most responsible for admission should be listed as the primary diagnosis. If a patient has a chronic medical condition that will be addressed during the hospital stay, that should be listed as an additional or secondary diagnosis. *Primary diagnosis: pneumonia. Secondary diagnosis: Type 2 diabetes.*

Condition

This reflects the patient's condition at the time of admission. If the patient has terminal cancer and is likely to die within a few hours, the condition should reflect that. Words commonly used to describe condition are *stable, unstable, guarded, critical, morbid,* and *comatose.*

Activity

Indicate the level of activity the patient is permitted to have. There are several activity orders commonly used; the condition of the patient (including mental alertness) and the overall health condition of the patient determine which order is most appropriate. Common activity orders include the following:

- up ad lib (the patient may be out of bed as he or she wishes)
- activity as tolerated (whatever the condition allows the patient to do)
- bed rest with bathroom privileges, abbreviated as BR with BRP (allowed out of bed to go to the bathroom; otherwise in bed)
- out of bed (OOB)
- ambulate a certain number of times a day
- ambulate with assistance
- non–weight-bearing

Vital signs

This order reflects how often the standard vital signs (T, P, R, and BP) should be obtained and will vary according to the patient's condition. Some hospitals have standing orders for vital signs depending on the type of unit or floor to which the patient is admitted. Critical or intensive care units almost always have their own standing orders. Some vital signs may be monitored continuously as the patient's condition dictates; for instance, BP and HR are moni-

AD CAVA DIMPLS

Admit: admitting physician and type of unit or hospital floor

Diagnosis: chief reason for the patient's admission

Condition: usually a one word description

Activity: level of activity allowed depending on age, diagnosis, medications, etc.

Vital signs: frequency with which vital signs should be obtained

Allergies: list any medication allergies

Diet: what type of diet patient is allowed

Interventions: IV therapy, respiratory therapy, etc.

Medications: medications related to reason for admission and any chronic medications the patient may be taking

Procedures: wound care, ostomy care, etc.

Labs: any laboratory or diagnostic tests needed

Special instructions: notify if certain parameters are exceeded, or conditional orders (if this occurs, then do this)

Figure 9–2. Admission orders mnemonic.

tored continuously in a patient who recently had a myocardial infarction. Typical orders for medical admissions are *VS q 8 hrs while awake* (if the patient is very stable and if it is not necessary to awaken a patient to obtain vital signs) and *VS q 4 hrs*.

Weight is generally obtained at the time of admission only and is not routinely included as part of vital signs. If it is necessary to monitor the patient's weight, write a specific order to do so. For instance, if a patient is admitted for congestive heart failure and has extensive edema and fluid retention, write an order to *weigh daily*.

Allergies

This is not actually an order but rather a specific notation of allergies the patient may have to any medication, food, or other substance. It is customary to include the specific agent the patient is allergic to and what reaction the

patient has to the agent. One way to note this is *Allergic to penicillin (rash) and aspirin (dyspnea).*

MEDICOLEGAL ALERT!
You should always document any allergies the patient has to medications, foods, or other substances, such as contrast medium. Latex allergy is especially important to document because of its use throughout the hospital. Any time you order a new medication, a diet, or a diagnostic study that uses contrast medium, you must check allergies to be sure you are not ordering something that is a known allergen. You should also avoid ordering any chemically related medications or substances. Doing so could be life-threatening for the patient and end your career.

Diet

The first step in determining which diet order to write is usually whether the patient should eat. If the patient is going to have surgery or a procedure that requires sedation and therefore carries a risk of aspiration, or if a patient is mentally not alert enough or physically able to eat and swallow, it might be safer for the patient not to receive any nourishment by mouth. The order for this is *NPO,* an abbreviation for the Latin, meaning *nothing by mouth.* If it is acceptable for the patient to eat, there are many diet orders that can be written. It is not possible to include all of them in this book. Hospitals have a dietary manual for more information, and consulting with a dietitian is also an option. See Table 9–1 to familiarize yourself with some of the more common types of diets for oral intake.

Interventions

This refers to interventions by nursing or other ancillary staff, such as physical therapy or respiratory therapy. One example of an intervention is *SVN (single volume nebulizer) with 0.5 cc Albuterol in 2.5 cc normal saline (NS) q 4 hrs.* Another example is *Physical therapist (PT) to instruct on bed to wheelchair transfers.* IV therapy is also considered an intervention. An order for an IV should specify the type of fluid and the rate of administration, such as D_5NS *(5% dextrose in NS) at 80 cc/hr.* (Consult the reference section for suggested readings related to principles of IV therapy.)

Medications

Make every effort to write medication orders that are precise and unambiguous.

MEDICOLEGAL ALERT!

Hospital errors have been the topic of much media attention. These errors are often related to how medication orders are written or how medications are administered. The possibility of an error related to medications during a hospital stay might be a source of anxiety for patients. The medical, nursing, and hospital pharmacy staff must work together to avoid such errors. The following common errors related to in-patient medication orders have been identified:

- Illegible writing, especially related to abbreviations
- Writing with a felt-tip pen
- Not specifying route of administration
- Not specifying dose
- Improper drug selection
- Ordering a medication for something other than its labeled use
- Not giving a medication at the time the dose is due
- Overdosing or subtherapeutic dosing
- Ordering a drug that interacts with something the patient is already taking
- Ordering a drug to which the patient is allergic
- Improperly modifying a medication order
- Absence or presence of trailing zeros
- Writing ampule or vial rather than strength

Table 9–1 **Common Diets for Oral Intake**		
Condition	**Dietary Intervention**	**Typical Order**
Diabetes	Calorie restriction and type of food (protein, vegetable, etc.); follows recommendations of the American Diabetes Association (ADA)	1400 calorie ADA diet
Hypertension	Sodium restriction	2 g Na$^+$ diet
Coronary artery disease or hypercholesterolemia	Fat and cholesterol restriction	Low-fat, low-cholesterol diet *or* National Cholesterol Education Program (NCEP) Step Two diet
Unable to chew well, ill-fitting dentures	Allow soft foods only	Soft mechanical diet

Always specify the name of the medication, the dose, the route of administration, and the frequency. It is common to write orders first for any new medications that are given for the condition necessitating hospitalization, then any medications taken before hospitalization that need to be continued, and then orders for any symptomatic medications.

Symptomatic medications are those that may or may not be needed. During a hospitalization, patients may experience sleeplessness, constipation, pain, nausea, etc. It is customary to anticipate these conditions and write orders upon admission so that medications are available to treat these symptoms as needed. Having these medications available if needed reduces discomfort for the patient and may prevent a phone call to you at 2 a.m. when a patient is having difficulty sleeping. These medications would be ordered on a PRN basis. They are given only as requested by the patient. If you write an order for a PRN medication, you always want to include what the medication is needed for. An order for *meperidine 25 mg IM (intramuscular) PRN* is open for interpretation. Although many would recognize that meperidine is a narcotic analgesic and would know that it is given to relieve pain, it is more appropriate to write the order as *meperidine 25 mg IM q 4 hrs PRN pain*. This prevents the medication from being administered for reasons other than pain and establishes a safe period in which the medication may be administered.

Procedures

Think about procedures that might be part of a patient's care. A patient with an indwelling urinary catheter needs daily catheter care, so you should write an order for that. Other procedures include wound care, ostomy care, decubitus care, dressing changes, and the like. Be sure to specify the frequency of procedures when writing orders.

Labs

It may be necessary to monitor certain laboratory values or obtain diagnostic studies as part of a patient's care. For instance, when a patient is on an anticoagulant medication, you monitor the bleeding time. If a patient develops fever and a cough, you might order a CXR. You should always have a rationale for ordering laboratory or other diagnostic studies. If a patient had surgery but had very little intraoperative bleeding, it is unnecessary to order *H&H* (hemoglobin and hematocrit) *q am;* you would not expect the values to change because there was little blood loss. When ordering radiographic studies, it is helpful to include what you are looking for as part of the order, *AP (anteroposterior) & lateral CXR to R/O atelectasis*. The radiologist interpreting the films will appreciate that information, and some hospitals and third-party payers require it.

MEDICOLEGAL ALERT!

Sometimes an order is written as a "stat" order, meaning it should be carried out urgently or immediately. If you write a stat order, be sure that there is an indication to do so, then follow up on the order in a timely manner. Suppose you order a stat H&H at 0730. At 0820, the results of the H&H are placed in the medical record, but you do not see the result until 1630 when you make afternoon rounds. If the level was low and required an intervention, such as a blood transfusion, and there is an adverse event because the intervention was not done in a timely manner, you could be found liable for any damages related to the adverse event. You could have to defend why you ordered a test to be done "stat" and then did not follow up on it until hours later.

Special instructions

This helps you remember any special instructions that should be given to the nursing staff. For instance, a diabetic patient will have blood glucose monitoring on a regular basis. You will want to know if the result comes back above or below a certain level, because that would indicate the need for a change in treatment. You would write an order to *Notify Dr. Williams if blood sugar is <100 mg/dL or >350 mg/dL* (deciliter). If a patient was admitted 2 days ago for an acute MI and now has new onset of atrial fibrillation, you want to be alerted to that fact. You should never assume that the nursing staff will automatically notify you of such developments. As a general rule, they probably would, but the burden of being aware of changes in the patient's condition and implementing treatment as needed is on the attending medical staff, not the nursing staff. Writing the order protects you as a clinician and helps to ensure the best treatment for the patient.

The Surgical Admission

We use a case study format to introduce you to documentation for a surgical admission. The patient for the case study is Mr. William Jensen. Mr. Jensen has recently been diagnosed with adenocarcinoma of the colon and is being admitted to the hospital for an elective surgical procedure. An admission H&P for Mr. Jensen is shown in Figure 9–3. To become familiar with this patient, you should read the entire H&P before continuing any further. You will analyze and write several medical records related to Mr. Jensen's hospital stay.

Application Exercise 9.1

Referring to the information found in the H&P for Mr. Jensen (Figure 9–3), write an admit note in the space provided. Label it as an admit note, record the date and time of the entry, and provide the information as indicated in the above paragraph. Admit notes for surgical admissions do not vary greatly from those for medical admissions. The plan of treatment is the surgical procedure the patient is scheduled to have.

_____

_____

_____

_____

_____

Once you have completed your admit note, compare it with Example 9–2 below. How did you do?

EXAMPLE 9–2: ADMIT NOTE FOR MR. JENSEN

Mr. Jensen is a 67-year-old Caucasian man who has colon cancer. Mr. Jensen originally presented with complaints of fatigue and on workup was found to have blood in the stool. Colonoscopy revealed adenocarcinoma. Past medical history is significant for hypertension and hypercholesterolemia. He is taking Cardizem 120 SR once daily and Mevacor 20 mg once daily. He is allergic to sulfa medications, which causes a rash. Laboratory studies done at time of admission reveal that the CBC is normal; the chemistry panel reveals triglyceride of 178; LDL of 208; total cholesterol of 267; CEA of 17; otherwise WNL. CXR shows borderline cardiomegaly but no effusion. The EKG is WNL. Mr. Jensen will be admitted for elective right hemicolectomy. Routine preoperative orders are written. H&P done and dictated.

Perioperative Orders

When a patient is admitted for surgery, the initial preoperative orders are in effect until the patient goes to surgery. Once the surgery has been performed, the patient is essentially readmitted, and a new set of postoperative orders must be written. Preoperative orders for Mr. Jensen are shown in Figure 9–4. We will use the same mnemonic provided earlier, AD CAVA DIMPLS, to write the postoperative orders for Mr. Jensen.

Admit: The patient is typically admitted to the surgeon.

Diagnosis: The postoperative admitting diagnosis is usually the surgical procedure. For instance, Mr. Jensen's admitting diagnosis could be written as _hemicolectomy_. You may see _S/P hemicolectomy_, meaning "status post."

Condition: Condition refers to how the patient is immediately after surgery when the postoperative orders are written.

Activity: When writing the activity order, keep in mind that postoperative patients usually require at least some narcotic pain relief, which may impair judgment or function. Safety precautions may be indicated, such as _side rails up at all times_ or _ambulate only with assistance_. To prevent complications associated with immobility, patients are usually encouraged to be out of bed immediately postoperatively, but the activity level must take into consideration the type of surgery the patient has had. An activity order for Mr. Jensen could be _OOB TID_ (three times a day) _with assistance_.

Vital signs: In the immediate postoperative period, vital signs are obtained progressively. A common postoperative order would be _VS q hr × 4_; if stable, then _q 2 hrs × 4, then q 4 hours_. An order such as this reflects the possibility that a patient's condition might change in the immediate postoperative period and that more frequent assessment is needed initially, but if the patient's vital signs remain stable, less frequent assessment is permitted.

Allergies: Any allergies should be noted in the orders.

Diet: Surgical patients usually have special dietary needs in the preoperative and postoperative periods. The type of surgery and the type of anesthesia usually determines the type of diet ordered. As a general rule, patients who have general anesthesia should be NPO for 8 hours or more before surgery to avoid gastric distention and to reduce the risk of postoperative vomiting

PATIENT NAME: *William R. Jensen*   ADMIT DATE: xx/xx/xx
SEX: *male*   ADMITTING PHYSICIAN: *David K. Sanders, MD*
DOB: xx/xx/xx   MEDICAL RECORD #: *35-87-26*
CHIEF COMPLAINT:
"I have cancer, and I'm going to have surgery".

HISTORY OF PRESENT ILLNESS:

This is a 67-year-old Caucasian male who was referred to me by his primary care physician, Scott Vernon, MD after being diagnosed with colon cancer. Mr. Jensen initially presented to Dr. Vernon's office with complaints of fatigue and "feeling weak". During a routine workup, he was found to have hemoccult positive stool. At that time, Mr. Jensen was referred to a gastroenterologist, Michael Bennett, MD. Dr. Bennett performed a colonoscopy on Mr. Jensen, and found several suspicious polypoid lesions at the right hepatic flexure area. Biopsies were obtained and sent to pathology. Pathology reports indicate adenocarcinoma, with staging of $T_3 N_0 M_0$ (formerly Dukes B_1). Dr. Vernon and Dr. Bennett consulted, and they referred Mr. Jensen to me for surgical evaluation. I saw Mr. Jensen in my office on xx/xx/xx and discussed with him options for treatment. I recommended that we proceed with a right hemi-colectomy. Mr. Jensen was agreeable with this, and is admitted now for elective surgery.

PAST MEDICAL HISTORY:

MEDICAL: Mr. Jensen has a history of hypertension, hypercholesterolemia, and left inguinal hernia.

SURGICAL: Mr. Jensen has had repair of a torn rotator cuff, right shoulder, (Dr. Rodriquez, Sante Fe, NM) approximately 24 years ago. He has also had a left inguinal herniorraphy approximately 15 years ago (Dr. Simmons, Tucson, AZ). He has not had any blood transfusions.

MEDICATIONS: Cardizem 120 SR, once daily; Mevacor 20 mg once daily. Occasional acetaminophen.

ALLERGIES: Mr. Jensen states an allergy to **SULFA DRUGS** and breaks out in a rash when he takes anything containing sulfa.

HEALTH MAINTENANCE: Last complete physical two years ago. Mr. Jensen did get a flu vaccine September 2003, and his last tetanus immunization was in 2001.

FAMILY HISTORY:

Father is deceased, age 74, complications of COPD and alcoholism. Mother deceased, age 70, breast cancer. One sibling, age 69, who also has hypertension. One sibling, deceased, age 20 secondary to gunshot wound sustained in combat. Three children, alive and well, no significant medical history. Negative family history of diabetes, myocardial infarction. Positive family history of cancer, hypertension/CAD, and COPD.

Figure 9–3. History and physical (H&P).

SOCIAL HISTORY:

Mr. Jensen is a retired electrician. He is married, and lives in a single story home with his wife. They have three adult children who all live nearby. Mr. Jensen smokes a pipe about 3 times a week. He does not drink alcohol or use any recreational drugs. He is still active, and walks approximately two miles 4 of 7 days per week. He also bicycles occasionally.

REVIEW OF SYSTEMS:

GENERAL: Easily fatigued, feels weak. Denies any near-syncope or lightheadedness.

HEENT: Denies recurrent headaches. No hearing loss or ringing in ears. He has worn glasses since 1985. Denies loss of vision, double vision, or history of cataracts. Denies nasal drainage. Denies chronic or recurrent sore throat.

RESPIRATORY. He denies SOB, DOE, or hemoptysis. Last chest x-ray was 2 years ago.

CARDIOVASCULAR. Specifically denies chest pain, angina, and pleuritic pain. Denies any heart palpitations or irregularities in rhythm. No history of heart murmur. Denies peripheral edema.

GASTROINTESTINAL. Some "indigestion" self-treated with liquid antacid. Rarely occurs more than twice per week, and has always been relieved with antacid. Denies any difficulty swallowing or chewing. No change in bowel or bladder habits. No weight change in past 5 years.

GENITOURINARY: Denies any penile discharge or erectile dysfunction. No dribbling, incontinence or loss of force of stream.

MUSCULOSKELETAL: Denies any joint swelling or loss of range of motion.

PSYCHIATRIC: Denies any depression or mood swings. Denies any history of mental illness, drug, or alcohol abuse.

HEMATOLOGIC: Denies easy bruising or bleeding from gums.

ENDOCRINE: Denies heat or cold intolerance, excessive thirst or urination, tremors.

PHYSICAL EXAM

VITAL SIGNS: BP 142/80; P 86 and regular, R 16 and regular; Temp 97.8 orally. His current weight is 174 pounds.

GENERAL: Mr. Jensen is a well-developed, well nourished Caucasian male who is alert and cooperative. He is a good historian and answers questions appropriately.

HEENT: Head normocephalic, atraumatic. Pupils equal and reactive to light. Wearing glasses. TMs unremarkable. Nose patent bilateral. No polyps noted. Oropharynx without erythema or exudate. Buccal mucosa intact without lesions. Patient is normally edentulous, wearing dentures presently.

Figure 9–3. History and physical (H&P).

NECK: Supple, full range of motion. No thyromegaly. No carotid bruits. No masses palpated. No tracheal deviation noted.

CHEST: Breath sounds clear to auscultation in all lung fields. Respiratory excursion symmetrical. Heart regular rate and rhythm. No murmurs, gallops, or rubs.

ABDOMEN: Soft, non-tender. No masses or organomegaly. Bowel sounds physiologic in all four quadrants. There is no guarding or rebound noted.

RECTAL/GU: Prostate non-tender, not enlarged. Stool guaiac positive. External genitalia exam reveals a circumcised male, both testes descended. No testicular or scrotal masses noted.

MUSCULOSKELETAL: Fully weight bearing. Full ROM all extremities. Well-healed surgical scars noted right anterior shoulder and left inguinal canal. No joint effusions, clubbing, cyanosis, or edema.

SKIN: Intact, no lesions or rashes noted. Turgor is good.

NEUROLOGICAL: CN II-XII grossly intact. Motor: +5/5 upper and lower extremities. Sensory intact to pinprick. Mood and affect appropriate to situation. DTRs intact and symmetrical.

LABORATORY DATA:

CBC: WBC 5800; Hct 48; Hgb 16. Peripheral smear shows normochromic, normocytic cells, differential unremarkable.

Chemistry: triglycerides 178; LDL 208; total cholesterol 267; CEA (carcinoembryonic antigen) of 17; otherwise WNL.

CXR: borderline cardiomegaly, no consolidations or effusions. UA: WNL.

PT, PTT (partial thromboplastin time): 12.4 and 31.

ECG: normal sinus rhythm with rate of 84. No ectopy, no ischemic changes.

ASSESSMENT:

1. Adenocarcinoma of the colon.
2. Hypertension, well controlled.
3. Hypercholesterolemia, fairly well controlled.

PLAN:

Mr. Jensen is admitted for a right hemicolectomy. Admission orders written. Will consult with Drs. Vernon and Bennett in the management of this patient. Routine postoperative care.

David K. Sanders, MD

DD: xx/xx/xx 0927

DT: xx/xx/xx 1132

Figure 9–3. History and physical (H&P).

xx/xx/xx 2030   1) Admit to Dr. Sanders, surgical floor

2) DX: colon cancer

3) Condition: good

4) Activity ad lib

5) Vital signs q shift

6) Allergic to SULFA

7) Regular diet now; NPO after midnight

8) Instruct on use of incentive spirometry

9) IV D_5 NS at 80cc/hr

10) Restoril 15 mg at hs PRN sleeplessness

11) Valium 5 mg IM on call to OR (operating room)

12) Hold routine meds at present

Signature, title

Countersignature

Figure 9–4. Preoperative orders for Mr. Jensen.

and aspiration. When a patient undergoes surgery involving the gastrointestinal tract, paralyzing agents are often used to prevent peristalsis during surgery. Various factors such as age, mobility, and overall health status affect how quickly bowel function returns after surgery. Patients are kept NPO until bowel function returns. Once bowel function resumes, indicated by the return of bowel sounds, the diet is advanced from liquids to solids as tolerated. Typically, the first diet order is *clear liquids*. If the patient is able to tolerate clear liquids without any nausea or vomiting, the diet is advanced to *full liquids*, then to a *regular diet* or any special diet indicated for specific medical conditions. Table 9–2 provides information about the liquids and foods allowed on clear and full liquid diets. Some practitioners might prefer to write an order to *advance diet as tolerated* and not specify when to advance the diet or what type of diet to follow, leaving the details to the judgment of the nursing or dietary staff.

Table 9-2	Diets Commonly Used in the Postoperative Period
Clear Liquid Diet	**Foods**
	Broth
	Gelatin
	Tea
	Apple juice, cranberry juice, grape juice
	Pedialyte
	Gatorade
	Clear sodas, such as lemon-lime or ginger ale
Full Liquid Diet	All the foods shown for clear liquid diet plus:
	Coffee
	Milkshake, ice cream, sherbet
	All soups
	Oatmeal, cream of wheat, grits, gravy
	Dark sodas, such as colas
	Orange juice, grapefruit juice, pineapple juice
Soft Diet	
	Oatmeal
	Mashed or baked potatoes
	Bananas
	Scrambled eggs
	Soft bread or rolls (not toasted)
	Applesauce
	Gelatin
	Puddings

Interventions: Like any patient who has had abdominal surgery, Mr. Jensen is likely to have shallow respirations postoperatively, which puts him at risk for pulmonary complications. To prevent such complications, an important intervention order for Mr. Jensen is *incentive spirometry* (ICS) *q 4 hrs while awake*. In some institutions, the nursing staff will instruct the patient on spirometry; in others, a respiratory therapist does this. Another important intervention is maintaining hydration and nutrition. Until adequate oral intake is possible, IV fluids should be administered. For Mr. Jensen, we will order *D_5NS @ 120 cc/hr*.

Medications: Mr. Jensen will require some medications. Medications administered orally are withheld until bowel function returns.

Symptomatic medications are indicated, especially for pain and nausea. Specify not only the name of the medication but also the dose, route, and frequency, and for any PRN medications, the indications for them. One analgesic used postoperatively is meperidine (Demerol). In this case, we write *meperidine 50 mg IM q 4 hrs PRN pain*. Some hospitals prefer the use of generic medication names, whereas others accept generic or trade names. Check with the hospital pharmacy to be sure which you should use. Another option for postoperative pain control would be patient-controlled analgesia (PCA). Using PCA, analgesia is delivered intravenously when the patient pushes a button that controls a pump dispensing the medication. Dose limits can be set on the pump to prevent an overdose. An antiemetic is usually ordered as a PRN medication. Nausea is fairly common in the postoperative period, and antiemetics can reduce nausea and prevent vomiting. Most antiemetics potentiate the action of narcotic analgesics, so they are frequently administered together. The analgesics and antiemetics should be ordered separately, however, so that they may be administered individually if both are not needed.

Once bowel function returns, Mr. Jensen's preoperative medications should be ordered. It is also desirable to change from parenteral analgesics to oral analgesics when the patient is able to tolerate oral intake. In fact, the patient's ability to tolerate oral food and medications and obtain effective pain relief from oral analgesics are often considered criteria for discharge.

Procedures: One procedure indicated for Mr. Jensen is *daily wound care*. Order *daily catheter care* if the patient has an indwelling urinary catheter.

Laboratory or diagnostic studies: Laboratory studies are not indicated for Mr. Jensen, because he did not have any significant abnormalities from the preoperative laboratory studies and because he did not have any significant blood loss during surgery.

Special instructions: Some special instruction orders might be prudent for Mr. Jensen. Because he has a history of hypertension and usually takes antihypertensive medication, you would want to know whether his blood pressure was elevated above an acceptable level. Likewise, development of a fever would be important, and you would want to be notified if that occurred. A complete set of postoperative orders for Mr. Jensen is shown in Figure 9–5.

xx/xx/xx   1) Admit to Dr. Sanders, surgical floor

0723   2) DX: S/P right hemicolectomy

                3) Condition: stable

                4) Bed rest

                5) VS q 1 hr × 4, if stable q 2 hrs × 4, if stable q 4 hours

                6) Allergic to SULFA

                7) NPO

                8) Incentive spirometry q 4 hrs while awake

                9) I&O (intake and output)

                10) D_5 $^1/_2$ NS 150 cc/hr

                11) Demerol 25 – 50 mg IM q 4 hrs PRN pain

                12) Phenergan 25 mg IM q 4 hrs PRN nausea

                13) Routine wound care

                14) Routine catheter care

                15) Notify if systolic pressure > 150 mm/Hg or HR > 130

                                        Signature, Title
                                        Countersignature

Figure 9–5. Postoperative orders for Mr. Jensen.

To reinforce abbreviations used in this chapter, please complete Worksheet 9.2 at the end of this chapter.

Chapter Summary

- A complete H&P should be performed and documented using standard format within 48 hours of admission.

- The admit note will provide a brief summary of the H&P until the completed transcribed record is placed in the chart.

- Admission orders should be written in a timely manner, using the mnemonic AD CAVA DIMPLS to remember what to include in the orders.

- The documentation related to a surgical admission will have certain special considerations and will differ somewhat from that of a medical admission.

- Refer to the numbered list in this text for tips on dictating hospital records.

- Remember, if it is not documented, it was not done!

Chapter 10

Documenting Daily Rounds and Other Events

The Daily Progress Note

Whenever a patient is in the hospital, the admitting physician or a designee must visit the patient daily. This is often referred to as "making rounds" or "rounding on a patient." The purpose of the daily visit is to see how patients are responding to treatment and to determine whether any new problems have arisen. The SOAP note format that you studied in Section 1 is frequently used to record information from the daily rounds. When documenting the SOAP note in the chart of a patient who has had a surgical procedure, it is customary to label the note as "POD (postoperative day) # ," indicating what number postoperative day it is. Subjective information includes the patient's comments or complaints and comments made by family members or health-care providers. Objective information includes vital signs, weight, general assessment, physical examination findings, laboratory or diagnostic study findings, intake and output (I&O), and medications or other therapies. Assessment indicates how the patient is progressing and the patient's response to therapies. The plan addresses any new problems or indicates any changes in the present care.

MEDICOLEGAL ALERT!

You may be responsible for rounding on more than one patient. Before making any entries in a patient's chart, take the time to verify that you have the correct chart. You should always check the name on the chart and check individual pages within the chart to be sure the patient identification data match the patient you want to document. Making an entry in the wrong chart could result in a variety of problems, ranging from mere inconvenience to something much more serious. A good practice is "make sure it's right before you write!"

Content of a Daily Progress Note

When you assess a postoperative patient during daily rounds, some basic questions must be answered: Is the patient getting adequate pain relief from the analgesic? Has bowel function returned? Can the activity level be advanced? Can the diet be advanced? Can any sutures, staples, tubes, or drains be removed? Are any laboratory, radiographic, or other diagnostic studies needed? Does the patient have any complaints or new problems? Are any consultations or special services needed? Is the patient nearing discharge? The answers to these questions should be documented in the daily progress notes.

You should also determine whether any postoperative complications have occurred. You can anticipate what complications might arise and then document enough information to convey to other providers that such complications have or have not occurred. Common postoperative complications include fever, urinary retention, fluid imbalance, and wound infection. More serious complications include hemorrhage, respiratory depression, and pulmonary or fat embolism. Fever is the most common postoperative complication and usually has one of four etiologies. You can remember these etiologies by thinking of wind, wound, water, and walk (the "four Ws," explained in Table 10–1). This will help you remember to assess the lungs, appearance of the wound, urinary status, and lower extremities. You will then document the pertinent positives or negatives related to each of these assessments.

Application Exercise 10.1

Write the S and O portions of a POD 1 progress note for Mr. Jensen, using the information below and the information in Table 10–2.

From your review of his chart, you determine that Mr. Jensen is NPO and on BR, has an order for an IM analgesic as needed, and has an IV and a urinary catheter. The most recent vital

Table 10-2 Physical Examination Findings for Mr. Jensen, POD #1

System	Findings
General	Awake, alert, cooperative
Chest	Respirations somewhat shallow, but breath sounds without any wheezing or rhonchi; heart rate and rhythm regular
Abdomen	Soft, nondistended; minimal tenderness to palpation around operative incision; small amount of serosanguineous drainage noted on dressing; wound edges dry and intact, and no erythema or warmth around the incision; no bowel sounds audible
Lower extremities	No calf tenderness or swelling, no erythema or increased warmth to touch, distal pulses intact and equal bilaterally

signs recorded for Mr. Jensen are BP 136/86, T 98.8°F, P 92, and R 16. The maximum temperature recorded since surgery is 99.1°F. Intake of 1870 cc is charted in the nursing notes with an output of 1710 cc. You speak with the nurse caring for Mr. Jensen today, who relates that he seemed to rest well last night and has not had any complaints today. You enter the room and interview Mr. Jensen. He states that he slept fairly well last night and has been getting adequate pain relief from the medication. He does not have any complaints. You note that the drainage bag connected to the urinary catheter contains 75 cc of clear yellow urine. You perform a physical examination, the results of which are shown in Table 10–2. After analyzing the subjective and

Table 10-1 The Four Ws of Postoperative Fever

Category	System	When Fever is Likely to Occur	Potential Problems	What to Assess
Wind	Respiratory	Within first 48 hours after surgery	Hypoventilation, atelectasis, pneumonia	Respiratory rate and effort, breath sounds
Wound	Integumentary	4th-7th day postoperatively	Wound infection, abscess	Amount and character of drainage, erythema, induration, increased tenderness at operative site
Water	Urinary	Anytime	UTI, sepsis	Fever, chills, flank pain, urgency, dysuria; amount, color, and smell of urine
Walk	Vascular	5th–14th day postoperatively	DVT (deep vein thrombosis)	Calf tenderness, swelling, warm to touch; Homan's sign

objective information on Mr. Jensen, your assessment is that Mr. Jensen is progressing as expected and that he does not have any new problems. The plan portion of the SOAP note also needs to be documented. You decide that the urinary catheter should be removed and that Mr. Jensen should increase his activity and begin ambulating.

Now write the A and P portions of the SOAP note, and then compare your daily progress note to the one in Figure 10–1.

◾ Daily Orders

Any time there is a change in the plan of care for a hospital patient, corresponding orders must be written to reflect that change. Remember that in Chapter 9 we said that an order stays in effect until another order is written to change it or cancel it. Once you have assessed the patient and recorded the daily progress note in the chart, you should write orders that reflect the changes addressed in your plan. You might want to refer back to Figure 9–5 to refresh your memory of the postoperative orders that are currently in effect for Mr. Jensen. Now, look at the plan portion of your SOAP note or the one shown in Figure 10–1. You will notice that an order should be written to remove the urinary catheter and another order to change Mr. Jensen's activity level. As with any entry on the order sheet, indicate the date and time, write the necessary orders, and then add your signature and title.

Date   POD #1

Time   0823

S: Mr. Jensen states that he rested fairly well last night. He has required pain medication every 4–5 hours and has had adequate pain relief. The nurse indicates that Mr. Jensen has been using the incentive spirometer every 4 hours when awake. He does not have any complaints at this time.

O: Vital signs: BP 136/86, P 92, R 16, temp is 98.8. Maximum temp since surgery has been 99.1. I & O is 1870 cc and 1710 cc. On exam, Mr. Jensen is awake, alert, and cooperative. Respirations are somewhat shallow, but breath sounds are without any wheezing or ronchi; heart rate and rhythm is regular. The abdomen is soft, non-distended; minimal tenderness to palpation around operative incision; small amount of serosanguineous drainage noted on dressing; wound edges are dry and intact, and there is no erythema or warmth around the incision. No bowel sounds audible. Lower extremities reveal no calf tenderness or swelling, no erythema or increased warmth to touch; distal pulses are intact and equal bilaterally. IV is infusing in the left lower arm. Urinary catheter in place with 75 cc of clear yellow urine in drainage bag.

A: S/P hemicolectomy, day 1. Progressing as expected without complications.

P: Remove catheter. May have BRP. Advance activity to OOB at least TID.

Signature, title.

Countersignature

Please note that the blank lines between sections of the SOAP note are for ease of reading only. When making an actual entry in the medical record, do not leave any blank lines.

Figure 10–1. First postoperative day progress note.

You may leave a blank line between this new set of orders and the previous set of orders, but do not leave any blank lines between the individual orders.

Your orders should read something like this:

xx/xx/xx 1) Discontinue catheter

0847   2) BRP

          3) OOB at least TID

                    Signature, Title

The second order, BRP, indicates that Mr. Jensen is now allowed out of bed to go to the bathroom. The third order indicates that he should be out of bed at least three times each day. All the other postoperative orders (Figure 9–5) are still in effect. When you write orders for an intervention, be sure to assess the patient's response the next day, and document that assessment in the progress note. For instance, in the orders above, an order was written to remove the urinary catheter. The next day when you round on Mr. Jensen, you want to see how he responded to removal of the catheter. Was he able to void after the catheter was removed? Did he experience any urinary retention? Your documentation should reflect how the patient responded to the intervention.

Application Exercise 10.2

Using the information below, write a POD 2 progress note and any orders necessary.

Mr. Jensen states that he rested fairly well last night. He has required pain medication every 4 hours. He was able to void after the catheter was removed. He experienced minor discomfort when he was out of bed but continues to have adequate pain relief. He denies any chest pain, DOE , or difficulty breathing. He denies any nausea or vomiting and states that he feels hungry. Continues to use the ICS every 4 hours when awake. He does not have any complaints at this time.

A review of the medical record indicates vital signs as follows: BP 152/90, P 98, R 20, T 99.2°F. Maximum T since surgery has been 99.7°F. I&O are 1855 cc and 1635 cc. On physical examination, Mr. Jensen is awake and cooperative. Respirations are nonlabored, and breath sounds are without any wheezing or rhonchi. Heart regular rate and rhythm, no murmur or ectopy. The abdomen is soft, nondistended; minimal

tenderness to palpation around operative incision. Dressing is dry. Wound edges are intact, and there is no erythema or warmth around the incision. Faint hypoactive bowel sounds heard throughout. No calf tenderness to palpation. No swelling or edema of lower extremities. Distal pulses are intact and equal bilaterally. IV is infusing in the left lower arm.

APPLICATION EXERCISE 10.2 ANSWER

Here is one possible POD 2 note and orders for Mr. Jensen:

S: Mr. Jensen states that he rested fairly well last night. He has required pain medication every 4 hours. He was able to void after the catheter was removed. He experienced minor discomfort when he was out of bed but continues to have adequate pain relief. He denies any chest pain, dyspnea on exertion, or difficulty breathing. He denies any nausea or vomiting and states that he feels hungry. He continues to use the incentive spirometer every 4 hours when awake. He does not have any complaints at this time.

O: Vital signs: BP 152/90, P 98, R 20, T 99.2°F. Maximum T since surgery has been 99.7°F. I&O are 1855 cc and 1635 cc. Mr. Jensen is awake and cooperative. Respirations are nonlabored and breath sounds are without any wheezing or rhonchi. Heart regular rate and rhythm, no murmur or ectopy. The abdomen is soft, nondistended; minimal tenderness to palpation around operative incision. Dressing is dry. Wound edges are intact, and there is no erythema or warmth around the incision. Faint hypoactive bowel sounds heard throughout. No calf tenderness to palpation. No swelling or edema of lower extremities. Distal pulses are intact and equal bilaterally. IV is infusing in the left lower arm.

A: Return of bowel function. BP elevated today but asymptomatic. Wound healing well.

P: Increase diet to clear liquids. Start on prehospital meds of Cardizem and Mevacor.

Activity as tolerated.

Orders to correspond to your plan would read as follows:

1. Increase diet to clear liquids

2. Activity as tolerated

3. Cardizem 120 SR one tablet po daily

4. Mevacor 20 mg one tablet po daily

MEDICOLEGAL ALERT!

Problems might arise when an intervention that should be done is omitted or when an intervention is performed longer than is necessary. An example is a patient who needs to have regular treatments with a bronchodilator, but the order is never written. The patient develops respiratory difficulty because an intervention was warranted but not done. There might also be problems if an intervention is done longer than necessary. An example of this is when a patient has a urinary catheter that could be removed, but such an order is not written. The catheter remains in place longer than necessary, and the patient develops a urinary tract infection. Always remember to assess on a daily basis what interventions are indicated and which ones may be discontinued.

Verbal Orders

During the course of a patient's hospitalization, a situation might arise that requires an intervention not already allowed for in the existing orders. It may be necessary to give an order verbally for a medication or for some specific intervention. Almost all institutions permit the use of verbal orders, but this should be limited to emergent or urgent situations, especially when the verbal order is for a medication. According to one study, confusion over the similarity of drug names accounts for approximately 25% of all reported medication errors. All the usual elements of a written medication should be included in a verbal order, such as name of the patient, drug name, dosage form, exact strength or concentration, dose frequency, route of administration, and specific instructions for use. Spell the name of any medication to avoid confusion or give both the generic and trade names. We also recommend that you speak numbers for dosing. For instance, a dose of 50 mg should be spoken as "fifty milligrams, five zero milligrams" to distinguish from other numbers that sound similar, such as 15. Instructions should be spoken clearly without abbreviations. Instead of saying "give one tab TID," you should say "give one tablet three times a day." The entire order should be repeated back to you for verification. The nurse taking the order should put it in writing as soon as possible. Verbal orders will be indicated as such in the medical records and should be countersigned by the prescriber as soon as possible.

Other Types of Documentation

In addition to admitting and rounding on patients daily, other events might occur in the care of the hospitalized patient that will have to be documented. Procedure, operative, and delivery notes are discussed in the following sections. Discharge summaries, discharge orders, patient elopement, and a patient leaving the hospital before discharge are discussed in the next chapter.

Procedure Note

The purpose of the procedure note is to document the performance of a procedure. The usual format includes the following elements:

- Name of the procedure
- Indication for the procedure
- Consent (if required, including risks and benefits, potential complications, and name and relationship of person giving consent)
- Anesthesia (if applicable)
- Details of the procedures
- Findings (if relevant)
- Complications

Suppose that, while he was in the hospital, Mr. Jensen fell and sustained a laceration to the scalp. You are called to evaluate him. After examination, you determine that the laceration requires closure. After the laceration is repaired, you document the procedure. An example of a complete procedure note for a laceration repair is shown.

xx/xx/xx   Procedure Note
1845   Procedure: Laceration repair
               Indication: 2 cm full thickness laceration of the right occipital area.
               Consent: Discussed with Mr. Jensen the need for laceration repair; possible complications of infection, bleeding; oral consent given by Mr. Jensen.

Anesthesia: Local with 1% lidocaine with epinephrine
Procedure: The area was prepped and draped in the usual sterile fashion. After local anesthesia, the wound was explored; no foreign bodies or step-offs were palpated. The wound was cleansed with Hibiclens and sterile water. The laceration was repaired with 3.0 nylon suture with a total of 4 interrupted sutures. Good approximation and hemostasis was achieved. Topical antibiotic ointment was applied.
Complications: None
Signature, title

MEDICOLEGAL ALERT!

The issues related to consent are complex. Consent is not merely a form that needs to be completed; obtaining the patient's consent means obtaining the patient's authorization for diagnosis and treatment. It is the responsibility of the physician or the physician's representative to discuss with the patient the indications for a procedure, the risks and benefits associated with the procedure, and any alternative forms of treatment. Courts have consistently held that it is not the responsibility of the hospital or healthcare organization or any of the employees to obtain consent. The person making the consent decision must be legally and actually competent and must be informed. A potential pitfall exists when there is more than one physician attending a patient and there may be confusion about which physician is responsible for obtaining consent. Generally, the burden to obtain consent rests with the person who will be performing the procedure for which consent is necessary. State laws may regulate who is responsible for obtaining consent and who may give consent. You are encouraged to consult the references provided at the end of this section for more information regarding consent.

Full Operative Report and Operative Note

Two entries related to the actual surgical procedure may appear in the chart. One is the full operative report, dictated by the surgeon, which provides details of the procedure. The other is a brief operative note that is documented in the chart immediately after surgery and remains part of the medical record even after the full operative report is placed on the chart. The usual format for the brief operative note includes many of the same components of the procedure note discussed above, but more detail is usually necessary. An operative note should contain the following information:

- Date of procedure
- Name of procedure
- Indication: reason for the procedure
- Surgeon
- Surgical assistants, if any
- Anesthesia: local, general, regional; name of anesthesiologist
- Preoperative diagnosis: presumptive diagnosis before surgery
- Postoperative diagnosis: most likely diagnosis based on surgical findings
- Descriptions
  1. Specimens: what tissue was removed and what studies were done
  2. Estimated blood loss (EBL)
  3. Drains: types of drains, if any, and where placed
- Complications, if any (such as a nicked artery, punctured bowel, or complications from anesthesia)
- Disposition

Application Exercise 10.3

The complete operative report for Mr. Jensen, dictated by the surgeon, is shown in Figure 10–2. Use the information from this report to compose a brief operative note in the space provided.

Date of procedure: _____

Name of procedure: _____

Indication: _____

Surgeon: _____

Surgical assistant: _____

Anesthesia: _____

Preoperative diagnosis: _____

Postoperative diagnosis: _____

Date of Procedure: xx/xx/xx

Procedure: Right hemicolectomy

Indication: adenocarcinoma diagnosed by tissue biopsy

Surgeon: D. K. Sanders, MD

Surgical Assistant: D. Sullivan, PA-C

Anesthesia: general, by P. Bartlett, MD

Preoperative Diagnosis: Adenocarcinoma, right colon

Postoperative Diagnosis: Adenocarcinoma, right colon

Description: Under endotracheal anesthesia, the patient's abdomen was prepped and draped. A midline incision was made. The liver was normal, except for a small cyst of the lateral aspect of the left lateral segment. The stomach, spleen, small bowel, and retroperitoneum were normal. There were no stones in the gallbladder. The colon was remarkable for a mass in the right colon. The right colon was mobilized and the ureter identified and preserved. The gastrocolic ligament was divided along its right side. The ileocolic vessels were transected near their takeoff from the SMA, and ligated with absorbable suture. The remaining mesentery was divided between clamps and ligated. The bowel ends were transected using a stapler. The resection included the right branch of the middle colic artery, and resection margins were in the distal ileum and transverse colon. Two tissue samples were obtained, one from the distal ileum and one from the transverse colon. An ileotransverse colostomy was performed using staples. The mesenteric defect was closed with staples. Hemostasis was checked and the incision was irrigated. The fascia was closed with a single layer of running #1 PDS. The subcutaneous tissues were irrigated, and the skin was closed with Vicryl. Estimated blood loss was 80 cc.

Complications: none

Disposition: The patient was transferred to the post-anesthesia care unit in stable condition.

Figure 10–2. Complete operative report.

Description: _____

Complications: _____

Disposition: _____

APPLICATION EXERCISE 10.3 ANSWERS

Here is one way the operative note for Mr. Jensen could be documented.

Date of procedure: xx/xx/xx
Name of procedure: Right hemicolectomy
Indication: Adenocarcinoma of the colon
Surgeon: D. Sanders, MD
Surgical assistant: D. Sullivan, PA-C
Anesthesia: General
Preoperative diagnosis: Adenocarcinoma, right colon
Postoperative diagnosis: Adenocarcinoma, right colon
Description: No unexpected findings, no evidence of metastasis, two tissue samples obtained for pathology; EBL 80 cc
Complications: None
Disposition: To recovery in stable condition

Delivery Note

A delivery note is used to document the outcome of an obstetrical admission. In many hospitals, the physician in attendance at the time of delivery is responsible for dictating a complete delivery note. This brief note serves much the same function as the brief operative note; to document the delivery in the medical record until the dictated note can be transcribed and put on the chart.

The key information that should be provided in a delivery note includes:

- Type of delivery (vaginal, cesarean, etc.)
- Estimated gestational age of the fetus
- Viability of the fetus
- Sex of the fetus
- Apgar scores at 1 and 5 minutes (see Table 10–3 for criteria for Apgar score)
- Weight of the fetus
- Delivery of the placenta, including number of vessels in the umbilical cord and whether the placenta was intact
- If any lacerations or episiotomies, what extent and how repaired
- Estimated blood loss
- Condition of mother immediately after delivery
- An example of a delivery note is provided here.

xx/xx/xx Delivery note:
1028 Normal, spontaneous vaginal delivery (NSVD) of a full-term viable male infant, Apgars of 7 and 9. Weight 7 pounds, 2 oz., delivered over a second-degree central episiotomy. Intact placenta expelled spontaneously, three-vessel cord. No vaginal, cervical, or external genital lacerations. Episiotomy repaired with 2.0 chromic. EBL of 40 cc. Patient in good condition, no complications.

To reinforce the content and abbreviations used in this chapter please complete Worksheets 10.1 and 10.2 at the end of this chapter.

Table 10–3 Apgar Scoring Criteria*

Clinical Sign	CRITERIA FOR ASSIGNED POINTS		
	0 points	**1 point**	**2 points**
Heart rate	Absent	<100	>100
Respiratory effort	Absent	Slow and irregular	Good; strong
Muscle tone	Flaccid	Some flexion of the arms and legs	Active movements
Reflex irritability (reaction to suction of nares with bulb syringe)	No response	Grimace	Crying vigorously, sneeze, or cough
Color	Blue, pale	Pink body, blue extremities	Pink all over

*Score of 0–4 at 1 minute after birth indicates severe depression, requiring immediate resuscitation; score of 5–7 indicates some nervous system depression, and score of 8–10 is normal. Score of 0–7 at 5 minutes after birth indicates high risk for subsequent central nervous system and other organ system dysfunction; score of 8–10 is normal.

Chapter Summary

- A daily progress note should be documented for each day of the patient's hospital stay, indicating the patient's response to treatment.

- Anticipate what complications might occur and document the pertinent positives or negatives related to each possible complication.

- If a patient develops fever postoperatively, think of the 4 Ws: wind, wound, water, walk.

- Any time the plan calls for a change in the present care, be sure to write an order reflecting that change.

- When any intervention is done, assess and document the effects of that intervention.

- Consent is more than a form, and proper disclosure of risks and benefits of a procedure and alternatives to the procedure should be provided to the patient before the consent form is signed.

- The brief operative note serves as a summary of the surgery until the full operative report is dictated, transcribed, and placed in the chart.

- Remember: if it is not documented, it was not done!

Chapter 11

Discharging a Patient

Discharge Orders

In Chapter 9, we saw that specific orders are written when a patient is admitted to the hospital. Likewise, specific orders are written at the time of discharge. Let's refer again to Mr. Jensen, and write discharge orders for him.

Disposition

The first discharge order usually indicates the disposition, or where the patient will go when discharged. The patient might go home or might be transferred to another facility such as an extended care or rehabilitation facility. In the case of Mr. Jensen, he will return home because he does not require specialized care. The first order will read *Discharge to home.*

Activity Level

The patient's activity level should be specified in the discharge orders. Mr. Jensen has an abdominal incision, so he should not do any heavy lifting or straining in order to prevent dehiscence of the wound. An order that says *Avoid heavy lifting* is vague, and the patient is usually not in the position to determine how much weight is too heavy. It is usually best to give a specific weight limit. A fairly low weight is advised for Mr. Jensen; 20 pounds is the maximum he should lift at this time, although some surgeons might limit the weight to 10 pounds.

Mr. Jensen has a surgical incision, so activity

orders should include care of the wound or specific instructions related to the wound. The wound can get wet but should not be immersed in water. Therefore, an order should specify *May shower but no tub bath or swimming.* Mr. Jensen will need to continue wound care at home. Instead of writing out the specific wound care orders, it is customary to write an order for the nursing staff to *Instruct on wound care.*

Diet

Consider what type of diet the patient should have at home. Ideally, the patient's diet has been advanced during the hospital stay to the same that it was before hospitalization. Mr. Jensen has a history of hypertension and hypercholesterolemia, so the diet order should reflect the need for a special diet. A reasonable order for Mr. Jensen is *Low-fat, low-cholesterol diet.*

Medication

Just as you had to write orders for medications while the patient was hospitalized, the discharge orders should indicate what medications the patient will continue after discharge. First, consider what prehospital medications the patient was taking. In Mr. Jensen's case, he was taking Cardizem 120 SR and Mevacor. Because these medications treat chronic conditions that he still has, they should be continued. The order is written: *Continue usual dosages of Cardizem SR and Mevacor.* Next, consider what medications might be indicated related to the reason for the hospitalization. Mr. Jensen had major abdominal surgery and is likely to need some pain medication after discharge. Usually, the same oral analgesic that was given in the hospital will be continued at home because its efficacy has been established, and the patient has been tolerating it without any problems. A prescription should be written for any medications the patient has not taken previously, so you will need to write a prescription for an analgesic (prescription writing is discussed in Section 4). Finally, consider whether other medications, prescription or over-the-counter, are needed. Some medications that may be needed include stool softeners, hypnotics, and nonsteroidal anti-inflammatory medications for mild to moderate pain. Be sure to write a prescription for any medications that are not available over-the-counter.

Follow-Up Care

Follow-up care should also be part of the discharge orders. Specify when and by whom the patient will be seen. Mr. Jensen will see the surgeon, Dr. Sanders, 1 week from the time of discharge for wound evaluation, removal of staples or sutures, and a routine postoperative check-up. The written order would say: *Follow-up with Dr. Sanders in 1 week.* Follow-up care should also include special instructions for the patient, such as notifying Dr. Sanders if any symptoms of complications occur. You should specify what symptoms should be reported, because the patient might not realize the importance of certain symptoms. Think of what postoperative complications might occur and what symptoms might be associated with those complications. Any patient who has had major abdominal surgery will be at risk for developing wound infection, pneumonia, deep vein thrombosis, or pulmonary embolus. Symptoms that correspond to these conditions include fever, redness or increased pain at the incision site, difficulty breathing, and pain in the leg. "Fever" is somewhat subjective (just like "heavy lifting" discussed earlier), so it is usually best to state a specific temperature that would be of concern. A typical order reads: *Notify Dr. Sanders of temperature greater than 100.5°F, redness or increased pain at incision site, cough, difficulty breathing, or pain or swelling of the leg.*

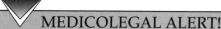

MEDICOLEGAL ALERT!

Failure to provide adequate follow-up instructions is one of the leading causes of litigation against healthcare providers. The provider has the responsibility to anticipate what complications the patient might develop and to educate the patient on the signs and symptoms that could indicate such a complication. Patients cannot be expected to know what signs or symptoms need to be reported. Your follow-up instructions and the documentation of such instructions should be as specific as possible. It is a good idea to verify that the patient has understood the follow-up instructions by asking the patient to repeat back to you what he or she has heard about the follow-up instructions. When you do this, you should document that the patient seemed to understand follow-up instructions. It is also recommended that you provide written follow-up instructions as well, because the patient is not likely to remember everything you said verbally. You should also include family members or others who may be caring for the patient after discharge and document who, besides the patient, received follow-up instructions.

A summary of what is included in discharge orders is shown in Figure 11–1. The entire set of discharge orders for Mr. Jensen would be as follows:

1. Discharge to home

2. No lifting >10 pounds, no exercising or strenuous activity

3. May shower but no tub bath or swimming

4. Instruct on routine wound care

5. Low-fat, low-cholesterol diet

6. Continue Cardizem SR and Mevacor at home

7. Vicodin 1 or 2 tablets po q 4 hrs PRN moderate to severe pain

8. Ibuprofen 600 mg po q 6 hours with food PRN mild to moderate pain

9. Colace 100 mg po twice daily for 1 week to prevent constipation

10. F/U with Dr. Sanders in 1 week

11. Notify Dr. Sanders if T >100.5°F, redness or increased pain at incision site, cough, difficulty breathing, or pain in legs

- Disposition (where the patient will go after discharged from hospital)

- Activity with specific instructions

- Diet

- Medications, including pre-hospital medications that should be resumed and any new medications

- Follow up instructions (when and who)

- Notification instructions (signs or symptoms that could signal complications)

Figure 11–1. Discharge orders.

Discharge Summary

The discharge summary is a synopsis of the patient's entire hospitalization and is usually required for any hospital stay longer than 24 hours. Often, members of the healthcare team, insurance carriers or other third-party payers, and quality assurance personnel request a copy of the discharge summary. Most of the time, a discharge summary must be completed before the hospital can submit for payment. For these reasons, the discharge summary should be completed in a timely manner. Regulations for participating in federal reimbursement programs, for example, require that hospital records be completed within 30 days following the patient's discharge. The discharge summary is usually dictated, and transcribed copies are placed in the chart and sent to the admitting physicians and other consulting providers as indicated.

One sample format is provided here, and we will again refer to Mr. Jensen as we discuss the discharge summary. Check with your hospital to see what format is used for the discharge summary because there may be variation. The headings shown below (and in Figure 11–2) indicate what information should be part of the discharge summary:

- Date of admission
- Date of discharge
- Admitting diagnosis (or diagnoses)
- Discharge diagnosis (or diagnoses)
- Attending physician
- Referring and consulting physician (if any)
- Procedures (if any)

- Brief history, pertinent physical examination findings and pertinent lab values (at time of admission)
- Hospital course
- Condition at discharge
- Disposition
- Discharge medications
- Discharge instructions and F/U
- Problem list

The dates of admission and discharge are easily determined from the chart. The admitting diagnosis can be found in the initial admitting orders. The discharge diagnosis might be the same as or different from the admitting diagnosis or might include several different diagnoses. If you have not been following the patient on a regular basis, you may have to read through the entire chart to identify all the diagnoses. The discharge diagnosis should be the primary reason for hospitalization; secondary diagnoses will be listed as well. For Mr. Jensen, we list *S/P (no change after) hemicolectomy* as the discharge diagnosis, with secondary diagnoses of adenocarcinoma of the colon, hypertension, and hypercholesterolemia.

The admitting physician is the physician primarily responsible for the patient during the entire hospitalization. For a surgical admission, this is almost always the surgeon. For a medical admission, look at the admitting orders to determine who the admitting physician was. Any consulting physicians who were involved in the care of the patient and the patient's primary care physician usually appreciate having a copy of the discharge summary.

Any surgical procedures the patient had

Date of Admission

Date of Discharge

Admitting Diagnosis (or diagnoses): principal or presumptive reason for admission

Discharge Diagnosis (or diagnoses): actual or final reason for admission that was evident by the time of discharge.

Attending Physician

Referring and Consulting Physician (if any): list names of those who provided consultations for this patient during the course of hospitalization; if none, omit heading

Procedures (if any): if none, omit heading.

Brief History, Pertinent Exam Findings and Pertinent Lab Values: events leading up to hospitalization, pertinent PMH, pertinent exam findings at time of admission, and pertinent lab values at time of admission.

Hospital Course: narrative of the details of the daily progress of the patient and response to treatment.

Condition at Discharge: avoid one-word descriptions, state why patient is able to be discharged.

Disposition: where patient will go at time of discharge (home, extended care facility, etc.)

Discharge Medications: list pre-hospital medications as well as any medications added during hospitalization that patient will continue taking after discharge.

Discharge Instructions and Follow-up: include activity level, signs or symptoms of potential complications that patient should report, and when patient should be seen for follow-up.

Problem List: include discharge diagnosis, any pre-existing conditions or chronic problems, as well as any new problems patient developed while in hospital; indicate if active problem or resolved.

Figure 11–2. Discharge summary contents and brief description.

during the hospitalization should be listed under Procedures. Some diagnostic or therapeutic procedures would be listed as well, such as a coronary arteriogram, a bronchoscopy, or wound débridement. Minor procedures are rarely included here, such as insertion or removal of a drain.

The brief history, pertinent physical examination findings, and laboratory data are in the admission H&P. You should not repeat everything already documented in these sections; instead, highlight any pertinent findings that are connected with the reason for the current hospitalization. The goal is to summarize the information already on the chart.

For the history, include enough information to indicate why hospitalization was necessary. In the case of Mr. Jensen, it is appropriate to mention his initial presentation of fatigue, the finding of blood in the stool, and the subsequent diagnosis of adenocarcinoma. Pertinent findings from the past medical history, current medications, and allergies are customarily included in this section of the discharge summary. There were no significant findings from Mr. Jensen's physical examination; thus, it is permissible to state: *The physical exam findings were unremarkable.* Pertinent baseline laboratory data should be summarized. For a surgical admission, the H&H is usually included (even if normal) as well as any abnormal findings from chemistry studies, such as the CEA of 17 for Mr. Jensen. His hypercholesterolemia is a chronic problem, so you could include the total cholesterol and triglyceride values, but because this chronic condition was not likely to have had a significant effect on this hospitalization, it is not absolutely necessary to include these values. An abnormality that needed correction before surgery or that would significantly affect the patient's condition is included in the summary.

Hospital Course

The hospital course is the most important part of the discharge summary. It can also be the most difficult part to write. Up to this point, you have basically been summarizing information taken directly from the medical record. The hospital course narrative is still a summary of information that is already recorded, but the challenge is learning what to include and what to leave out. It takes practice in the art and science of medicine and documentation to develop a good idea

for constructing the hospital course narrative. Think of this section as the story of the course of events of the hospitalization. You basically summarize the daily progress of the patient and the patient's response to treatment as documented in the daily progress notes. A great deal of detail usually is not needed, but include enough information to avoid ambiguity or an incomplete record of the patient's hospital stay.

Application Exercise 11.1

Read the hospital course narrative for Mr. Jensen that is provided in Example 11–1.

EXAMPLE 11-1

Mr. Jensen underwent an elective hemicolectomy without complications. Routine postoperative care was ordered. On POD 1, his maximum temperature was 99.7°F; maximum heart rate was 98, and the blood pressure range was 102/70 to 138/86. He required IM pain medication about every 6 hours with adequate relief. Mr. Jensen did not have any specific complaints. On exam, no bowel sounds were heard, so he was kept NPO with IV fluids. The wound edges were dry and intact without any warmth to touch or redness. Homan's sign was negative bilaterally. On POD 2, the IV was discontinued, and Mr. Jensen was started on clear liquids, which he tolerated well. He was able to ambulate with assistance and did not have significant pain. Vital signs remained stable, and his physical exam was unchanged. On POD 3, the diet was advanced to full liquids, and Mr. Jensen's preoperative medications of Cardizem 120 SR and Mevacor were started. The pain medication was changed from IM to PO. On POD 4, Mr. Jensen's vital signs were all stable, the wound was healing as expected, and he was tolerating a regular diet. He was able to ambulate without assistance and felt to be ready for discharge.

Now try to answer the following questions: When did bowel sounds return? Did Mr. Jensen have effective pain relief from the oral analgesic? Did Mr. Jensen experience any postoperative complications?

APPLICATION EXERCISE 11.1 ANSWER

We could assume that bowel sounds returned on POD 2 because the diet was advanced from NPO to clear liquids, but this information is not specifically mentioned. There is no documentation of how Mr. Jensen tolerated the oral analgesic, nor is there any specific information about postoperative complications. You might guess that, because none are mentioned, none occurred, but it is always best to provide enough information so that other people reading the discharge summary do not have to guess or make assumptions.

The discharge summary should also include a specific statement of the patient's condition. You want to let others know why the patient is ready for discharge. You should try to avoid one-word descriptions such as *stable* or *improved*. In the case of Mr. Jensen, you could state: *Mr. Jensen is tolerating a regular diet, has adequate pain relief from oral analgesics, and is able to ambulate without assistance and to perform activities of daily living. Postoperative recovery progressing as expected without complications.*

The disposition indicates where the patient goes when leaving the hospital. If the patient is being transferred to another facility, this should be indicated. For Mr. Jensen, we could say: *Discharged home in care of wife*. The discharge medications, instructions, and follow-up were discussed in the previous section on writing discharge orders. List the medications, and document any specific instructions in this part of the discharge summary.

Some facilities require that a discharge summary include a list of all the patient's medical problems. This information is especially helpful to other providers who will be caring for the patient in the future, especially if the patient was managed by a specialist or hospitalist and will receive primary care from a different provider. The problem list includes the discharge diagnosis, any pre-existing diagnoses or chronic problems, and any complications or new problems that the patient had during hospitalization. It is also helpful to indicate whether the problem is an ongoing problem or if it has been resolved. The problem list for Mr. Jensen looks like this:

1. S/P hemicolectomy

2. Adenocarcinoma of the colon

3. Hypertension

4. Hypercholesterolemia

A discharge summary for Mr. Jensen is shown in Figure 11–3. After reading it, try to answer these questions: When did bowel sounds return? Did Mr. Jensen have effective pain relief from the oral analgesic? Did he experience any postoperative complications? What medications is Mr. Jensen to take at home? When is Mr. Jensen to see Dr. Sanders? A well-written discharge summary will answer most if not all questions a reader might have about the events of the hospitalization.

Patient Leaving Before Discharge

Two events requiring careful documentation on your part are patient elopement and patients leaving the hospital against medical advice (AMA). Patient elopement occurs when a patient leaves the hospital without being discharged. Patients usually do not tell the nursing staff or the medical staff they want to leave; they just leave. You have no chance to intervene or try to get the patient to change his or her mind and remain in the hospital. If a patient elopes, you should write a final note in the chart, indicating what date and time you were informed of the elopement and who notified you. You still complete a discharge summary. In the disposition part of the discharge summary, you state that the patient eloped. An elopement prevents you from giving specific discharge instructions and follow-up care information to the patient, and it is customary to document that in your discharge summary.

A patient may tell you of a desire to leave the hospital before being ready for discharge. If this occurs, you should notify the admitting physician immediately. You or the admitting physician should discuss with the patient the benefits of continued hospitalization and treatment and the risks the patient will encounter if he or she chooses to leave. If you advise a patient to remain in the hospital and he or she still chooses to leave, the patient is said to be leaving AMA. If competent to make decisions, the patient has the right to refuse treatment and leave the hospital. Most hospitals have a standard form that patients should sign, indicating that they have been informed of the benefits of remaining in the hospital and the risks of leaving. An example of such a form is shown in Figure 11–4. Even if the patient signs such a form, document your conversation with the patient, and be as specific as possible about what benefits and risks you discussed with the patient. If nursing staff, family members, or others witness the discussion, you should document their names and relationship to the patient, if applicable. If you are able to arrange follow-up care for the patient, document the

ADMITTING PHYSICIAN: David K. Sanders, MD

Date of Admission: XX/XX/XX   Date of Discharge: XX/XX/XX

Admitting Diagnosis:

1. Adenocarcinoma of right colon

2. HTN

Discharge Diagnoses:

1. S/P Right hemicolectomy.

2. Adenocarcinoma of the colon.

3. HTN well controlled.

4. Hypercholesterolemia, fairly well controlled.

Brief History of Present Illness:

Mr. Jensen is a 67-year-old Caucasian male who was referred to me after being diagnosed with colon cancer. The patient underwent a diagnostic colonoscopy with biopsies, and pathology report indicated adenocarcinoma with staging of $T_3N_0M_0$. After discussing with Mr. Jensen and his wife the types of treatment available, they both agreed to an elective right hemicolectomy.

PMH:

Medical hx includes HTN and hypercholesterolemia. Surgical history includes repair of right rotator cuff 24 years ago, and left inguinal herniorrhaphy 15 years ago. Current medications include Cardizem 120 SR qd and Mevacor 20 mg qd. Patient is allergic to sulfa drugs, which causes a rash.

Physical Exam:
General:

BP 142/80, P 86 and regular, Temp 97.8 orally. Current weight 174 pounds. WDWN male, A & O × 3

HEENT:

unremarkable

Neck:

supple, full ROM.

Figure 11–3. Discharge summary for Mr. Jensen. (Continued on the following page)

Chest:

Breath sounds without wheezing or crackles. Respiratory excursion symmetrical. Heart RRR without murmurs, gallops, or rubs.

Abdomen:

Soft, non-tender. No masses or organomegaly. Bowel sounds physiologic in all four quadrants. No guarding or rebound noted.

Rectal/GU:

Prostate non-tender, not enlarged. Stool guaiac positive. External genitalia exam reveals a circumcised male, both testes descended. No testicular or scrotal masses.

Musculoskeletal:

No clubbing, cyanosis, or edema. Distal pulses intact.

Laboratory:

CBC: WBC 5800; Hct 48; Hgb 16. Peripheral smear shows normochromic, normocytic cells, differential WNL. Chemistry panel shows triglycerides of 178; LDL of 208; total cholesterol of 267; CEA of 17; otherwise WNL. Chest x-ray: borderline cardiomegaly, no consolidations of effusions.

UA: negative

PT, PTT: 12.4 and 31.

ECG: normal sinus rhythm with rate of 84. No ectopy, no ischemic changes

Hospital course:

Right hemicolectomy was performed xx/xx/xx without complications. Intraoperative findings were consistent with adenocarcinoma with no evidence of metastatic disease. IV of D5 1/2 NS and Demerol for postoperative pain management. On POD #1, patient did not voice any complaints. Blood pressure was 138/88, heart rate 92 max, respirations 20 and shallow. Max temp of 99.4. On exam, good breath sounds in all lung fields, no wheezing or crackles. Heart RRR. Abd soft and non-distended. Incision dry and intact without erythema or drainage. No calf tenderness or swelling. Orders to discontinue catheter. On POD #2, patient remained afebrile, max temp of 98.8, all other vital signs stable, Breath sounds clear, heart RRR. Faint bowel sounds were heard throughout. Wound

Figure 11–3. Discharge summary for Mr. Jensen. (Continued on the following page)

healing well without signs of infection. IM analgesics discontinued, changed to oral Percocet. Restart pre-hospital meds. Diet advanced to clear liquids. On POD #3, patient reported good pain relief with po meds and tolerating pre-hospital meds without difficulty. No nausea or vomiting with liquid diet. Full liquid diet was tolerated well. Patient reports having bowel movement (BM) this morning. Remained afebrile and all vital signs stable. No complaints. Lung and heart exam unchanged. No abdominal tenderness. Wound edges dry without erythema. Patient returned to regular diet. By POD #4, patient still afebrile, VS were WNL, wound healing without complications and signs of infections, tolerating regular diet and meds without difficulty. Patient ready for discharge.

Discharge instructions:

Patient will follow up with Dr. Sanders in one week for suture removal and will follow up with Dr. Vernon in 3 weeks for continue care. Continue wound care as instructed. He may shower and get the wound wet, but should not take tub baths or swim. He should be on a low-cholesterol diet. Activity level limited to no lifting over 10 pounds, no pulling or straining, until appointment with Dr. Sanders. Patient to notify Dr. Sanders if he develops temp > 100.5°F, SOB, swelling in legs, leg pain, or severe abdominal pain, cramping, or rectal bleeding.

Medications:

Patient will continue Mevacor and Cardizem. Given prescription for Percocet 5 mg, 1-2 po q 4-6 hrs PRN pain. Mr. Jensen was advised not to drive, drink alcohol, or operate any machinery while taking the Percocet. He should also drink lots of water to help avoid constipation, and may take Colace 100 mg (OTC) if needed.

Figure 11–3. Discharge summary for Mr. Jensen. (Continued)

discharge instructions and follow-up care just as you would for any other patient.

To reinforce the content and abbreviations used in this chapter, please complete Worksheets 11.1 and 11.2 at the end of this chapter.

◾ Chapter Summary

- Discharge orders must be written when a patient is ready to leave the hospital.
- The discharge summary should provide a narrative of the events of the entire hospitalization, especially treatments and the patient's response to treatments.
- Discharge instructions should be specific, not vague or general.

- If a patient elopes, you will not have the opportunity to inform him or her of the risks of leaving prematurely or the advantages of remaining in the hospital. You will still be required to complete a discharge summary.
- If a patient informs you he or she wants to leave the hospital before you believe he or she is ready for discharge, you should notify the attending physician immediately. The risks of leaving and the benefits of staying in the hospital should be explained to the patient. If the patient still chooses to leave, he or she should sign the appropriate form.
- Remember: if it is not documented, it was not done!

Release Against Medical Advice
General Hospital

Number (Above) and Name

Patient Name _____

Date _____   Time _____   ☐ AM   ☐ PM

I understand that I am leaving the above facility against medical advice. I have
been informed of the risks associated with leaving the facility and, knowing
these risks, I wish to leave this facility. I assume full responsibility for my own
care and welfare.

By signing this form, I release the attending physician, the facility, and its personnel, from all liability for any adverse effects, which may result from my leaving against medical advice.

Patient Signature: _____

If the patient is unable to consent by reason of age or some other factor, state the
reasons _____
_____

Signature of legally authorized representative _____

Witness _____

Figure 11–4. Release against medical advice form.

Prescription Writing

■ Purpose

Prescription writing is an integral part of outpatient care services, and writing prescriptions is often a part of discharging a hospitalized patient. Section 4 teaches you how to write prescriptions and how to transmit them by telephone. This section discusses writing prescriptions for controlled and noncontrolled substances and identifies common errors made in writing prescriptions. It further discusses how providers can protect the Drug Enforcement Agency (DEA) number.

As you read this section, keep in mind that laws governing prescription writing vary among states. It is your responsibility as a practicing professional to know and follow your state's regulations. Regulations concerning what must be imprinted on a prescription pad, use of duplicate forms, quantity of controlled substances that may be dispensed, and so on, vary greatly.

■ Objectives

- Present the elements of prescription writing.
- Provide information for writing prescriptions for controlled and noncontrolled substances.
- Apply the principles of prescription writing to transmitting prescriptions by telephone.
- Discuss common errors made when writing a prescription.
- Present commonly used abbreviations and discuss dangerous ones that should be avoided
- Discuss ways to protect a provider's DEA number.
- Use the information presented in this chapter to complete worksheet exercises.

Chapter 12

Prescription Writing

Elements of a Prescription

Certain elements should be included in every prescription, whether it is for a noncontrolled or a controlled substance. The basic elements include the following:

- Date the prescription was written
- Prescriber identification
- Patient identification
- The inscription
- The subscription
- Signa
- Indication
- Refill information
- Generic substitution
- Warnings
- Container information
- Prescriber's signature.

A summary of these elements is shown in Figure 12–1.

A medication is defined as controlled or noncontrolled, based on its potential for abuse or addiction. Noncontrolled medications are those that have low or no potential for abuse or addiction. Controlled substances have moderately high or high potential for abuse or addiction and are classified into one of five categories or schedules. For this reason, these substances are sometimes referred to as "scheduled" drugs. Table 12–1 presents the categories of controlled substances as defined by the Controlled Substances Act of 1970.

Writing Prescriptions for Noncontrolled Medications

Prescriber identification: In many cases this is preprinted on a standard prescription form. This includes the name and title of the prescriber and the address and telephone number of the practice or institution. When the prescriber is a PA, some states require that the supervising physician's name be preprinted on the prescription form as well.

Patient identification: Includes the patient's name; address; age or date of birth; and, sometimes, weight. It is recommended, and in some states it is required, that you use the patient's legal name instead of a nickname. If you are unsure of the patient's legal name, ask to see a driver's license or an insurance card if available. This helps avoid confusion and correctly identifies the patient. There is generally an address line on the prescription form, but providers often do not provide this information. The pharmacist will be required to verify this information in some instances, such as when a prescription for a controlled substance is being filled. The date of birth is more commonly requested than the patient's age, because it allows more specific identification. When a prescription is written for a pediatric patient, you should include the patient's weight so the pharmacist can verify that the medication has been dosed appropriately.

Inscription: The name and strength of the medication. The strength is the amount that should be dispensed, such as a 50 mg tablet or 250 mg per 5 mL. Some medications come in many different strengths and forms (i.e., tablets

Date of Prescription

Prescriber's Information: name and title, office or institution name, address, and phone number, blank line for DEA number.

Patient's Information: legal name, age or date of birth, address, weight if necessary.

Inscription: name of drug and strength.

Subscription: information for pharmacist regarding dosage form and number of doses to dispense.

Signa: instructions to patients including, route of administration, how often to take, special instructions, or indication for medication.

Refill information: number of refills or length of time prescription may be refilled

Generic substitution: indicate if a generic form is permissible or if medication is to be dispensed as written.

Warnings: what adverse effects may be caused by the medication, such as drowsiness, feeling shaky, etc.

Container information: use of childproof containers is required unless specifically indicated to use non-childproof container.

Provider's signature and title.

Figure 12–1. Summary of prescription elements.

and liquids). If you are unsure which strengths and forms are available, you should consult a prescribing guide, pharmacology text, or medication reference book. It is not the total amount to be taken by the patient over the course of the prescription. Generic or trade names may be used. Avoid abbreviating names of medications to help reduce the possibility of error. There are exceptions for well-known medications; for instance, trimethoprim sulfamethoxazole is commonly abbreviated TMP/SMX.

Subscription: Provides information to the pharmacist on dosage form and number of units or doses to dispense. Instructions about the dosage form may be tablets, capsules, suspension, etc. If a liquid or semiliquid is to be dispensed, provide the quantity, such as how many milliliters of suspension or how many grams in a tube. The amount dispensed should be the amount needed to complete a course of treatment. For example, if a patient is to take a tablet twice a day for 10 days, the subscription, or

Table 12-1 Drug Enforcement Agency Classification of Controlled Substances*

Category	Comments
I	High potential for abuse. No accepted medical use.
II	High potential for abuse. Use may lead to severe physical or psychological dependence.
III	Some potential for abuse. Use may lead to low to moderate physical dependence or psychological dependence.
IV	Low potential for abuse. Use may lead to limited physical or psychological dependence.
V	Subject to state and local regulations. Abuse potential is low.

*As in the Controlled Substances Act of 1970. Drugs are categorized according to their potential for abuse; the greater the potential, the more severe the limitations on their prescription.

amount to dispense, would be 20 tablets. You will often see either #20 or *Disp: 20 tabs;* either is acceptable.

Signa or sig: Provides instructions to the patient on how to take the medication and should be as specific as possible. This should include the route; any special instructions, such as *take on an empty stomach* or *with food,* and how often to take. When the medication is prescribed on an as needed (PRN) basis, the reason for taking the medication should be included. Avoid writing vague or ambiguous instructions such as *take as directed* or *apply in usual manner.* Numerous studies have documented that patients usually do not remember all the information they are given during the course of a provider/patient encounter; therefore, it is necessary to provide instructions that are as detailed and accurate as possible to reduce the chance that the medication may be taken inappropriately.

Abbreviations: Are frequently used when writing the instructions. A list of common abbreviations is shown in Table 12–2. There is controversy whether abbreviations should be used. Some providers and pharmacists think writing out instructions, rather than using abbreviations, would reduce the chance of a medication error. The National Coordinating Council for Medication Error Reporting and Prevention has

identified several abbreviations that are particularly dangerous because they have been consistently misunderstood. These abbreviations are shown in Table 12–3. The Council recommends that these should never be used in prescription writing.

Indication: Including the indication for the prescription is mandatory in some states. Even when states do not require an indication, the Institute for Safe Medication Practices recommends including it for two reasons. First, many drugs have names that look and sound alike. Second, illegible writing may cause confusion or misinterpretation. Including the indication for the prescribed medication provides another safety check for the prescriber, the pharmacist, and the patient.

Refill information: Should be included on the prescription form. This can be written as the number of times a prescription may be refilled or a period during which the prescription may be refilled. Most states impose a 1-year maximum refill period. Patients taking medications for chronic conditions should be assessed at least annually, so it is not prudent to write medication refills for more than a year period. If the patient has prescription coverage as a benefit of an insurance plan, it is a good idea to consult the formulary for that insurance company to see whether the medication you want to prescribe is covered and whether there are regulations about how many can be dispensed in a certain period. Many companies will cover only a 1-month supply of medication at a time. It is usually of monetary benefit to the patient to

Table 12-2 Common Abbreviations Used in Prescription Writing

Latin	Abbreviation	Meaning
ante cibum	ac	before meals
bis in die	bid	twice a day
gutta	gtt	drop
hora somni	hs	at bedtime
oculus dexter	od	right eye
oculus sinister	os	left eye
per os	po	by mouth
post cibum	pc	after meals
pro re nata	PRN	as needed
quaque 3 hora	q 3 h	every 3 hours
quaque die	q d	every day

Table 12–3 Dangerous Abbreviations to Avoid*

Abbreviation	Intended Meaning	Common Error
U	unit	Mistaken for a 0 or a 4, resulting in overdose. Also mistaken for cc when poorly written
μg	micrograms	Mistaken for mg, resulting in overdose
Q.D.	Latin abbreviation for *every day*	The period after the Q has sometimes been mistaken for an I, and the drug has been given qid (four times daily) rather than daily
Q.O.D.	Latin abbreviation for *every other day*	Misinterpreted as Q.D. (daily) or Q.I.D. (four times daily); if the O is poorly written, it looks like a period or an I
SC or SQ	subcutaneous	Mistaken as SL (sublingual) when poorly written
TIW	three times a week	Misinterpreted as *three times a day* or *twice a week*
HS	half strength	Misinterpreted as the Latin abbreviation HS *(hour of sleep)*
cc	cubic centimeter	Mistaken as U (unit) when poorly written
AU, AS, AD	Latin abbreviation for *both ears, left ear, right ear*	Misinterpreted as the Latin abbreviation OU *(both eyes)*, OS *(left eye)*, OD *(right eye)*

*Adapted from National Coordinating Council for Medication Error Reporting and Prevention, 1996.

prescribe a medication that is covered by the insurance plan, but that should not be the only factor considered when deciding which medication to prescribe.

Dispense as written: Most prescription forms will allow you to indicate whether the medication should be dispensed as written (DAW) or whether substitution of a generic form of the medication is permitted (Figure 12–2). Generic medications usually offer considerable cost savings to the patient, and with few exceptions it is preferable to allow them to be substituted.

Warnings: The prescription should specify what, if any, warning labels should be attached to the medication package or vial. In most instances, the pharmacist filling the prescription will automatically affix the appropriate warnings listed in the prescribing information, but the provider should include this information on the form. This provides another safety check between the provider and the pharmacist.

In many states, the law requires that pharmacists dispense medications in child-proof containers. If the patient taking the medication is likely to have difficulty opening such a container (such as a patient with arthritic hands), indicate that a non–child-proof container should be used.

Signature: The provider's signature authenticates the prescription. On a prescription form, the signature should include the name and the title of the prescriber. Signatures can be unique and may identify people, much like fingerprints, but above all they should be legible. Figure 12–3 shows a completed prescription with all the elements labeled.

Writing Prescriptions for Controlled Medications

Two main differences between noncontrolled and controlled medications are the quantity dispensed initially and refills. State laws regulate the quantity of controlled medications that can be prescribed during a certain period. When writing out the quantity, spell out the quantity instead of writing it numerically, or do both, as shown in Figure 12–4. This helps prevent modification of the prescription. State laws also regulate the number of refills, if any, allowed for controlled substances. It is your responsibility as a provider to know these regulations.

Midwestern University
Primary Care Pediatrics
19555 N. 59th Ave.
Glendale, AZ 85308
Phone: 623-572-3000
Fax: 623-572-3400

James E. Meyer, MD
DEA # _____

Debbie D. Sullivan, PA-C
DEA # _____

Name: _____   Age: _____

Address: _____   Date: _____

Refill _____ times   Childproof Container: ☐ yes   ☐ no

_____   _____
Dispense as written   Substitution Permitted

Figure 12–2. Signature lines.

Midwestern University
Primary Care Pediatrics
19555 N. 59th Ave.

Prescriber's   Glendale, AZ 85308
Information   Phone: 623-572-3000
Fax: 623-572-3400

James E. Meyer, MD

DEA # _____

Debbie D. Sullivan, PA-C

DEA # _____

Patient   Name: *Jane Smith*   Age: *24*
Information
Address: *11527 N. 83rd ave.*   Date: *xx/xx/xx*

Inscription: *Augmentin 250mg   tabs*
Subscription: *Disp: 30*
Signa: *Sig: ÷ po TID × 10 days for infection*

Refill   Refill __∅__ times   Childproof Container: ☑ yes ☐ no   **Childproof**
Information   **Container**
Information

Signature   _____   _____
Lines   Dispense as written   Substitution Permitted

Figure 12–3. Completed prescription with elements labeled.

Midwestern University
Primary Care Pediatrics
19555 N. 59th Ave.
Glendale, AZ 85308
Phone: 623-572-3000
Fax: 623-572-3400

James E. Meyer, MD
DEA # _____

Debbie D. Sullivan, PA-C
DEA # _____*MS12345XX*_____

Name: *John Smith*_____   Age: *40*_____

Address: *2830 Palo Verde Ct.*_____   Date: *xx/xx/xx*_____

Tylenol # 3 tabs
Disp: 10 (ten)
Sig: ÷ tab po q 4 hrs PRN pain

Refill *∅* times   Childproof Container: ☑ yes   ☐ no

_____   _____*DSullivan PAC*_____
Dispense as written   Substitution Permitted

Figure 12–4. Quantity to dispense-controlled substance.

MEDICOLEGAL ALERT!

According to some studies, up to 25% of ambulatory patients experience adverse medication events. Up to 6% of these adverse events could have been reduced or prevented altogether. Many preventable events involve prescribing a medication to which the patient has a known allergy. Before writing any new prescription for a patient, always ask about allergies to any medications, and prescribe accordingly. Sometimes, when asked about medication allergies, patients may describe what sounds like side effects of a medication rather than describing a true allergic reaction. If you have any doubt whether a patient is truly allergic to a medication, always err on the side of caution and do not prescribe it if there is even a remote chance the patient had an allergic reaction in the past. You should always consider what medications the patient is already taking, and determine the likelihood of drug interactions. Sometimes, the benefit of prescribing a specific medication may outweigh the possible risk of a drug interaction or side effect; document in such a way that reflects that you are aware of possible side effects or drug interactions but that you believe the medication still to be the most appropriate treatment for the patient's condition.

Telephone Transmission

Some states allow for transmitting prescriptions verbally via telephone for noncontrolled substances. The same elements that are represented on written form should be included verbally when a prescription is telephoned to the pharmacy. In some states, a pharmacy technician may receive an order to refill a prescription, but most states require that a licensed pharmacist receive an order for a new prescription. When telephoning the order, be sure to identify yourself, and provide your title. Provide the office setting or institution information, especially the phone number, in case someone at the pharmacy needs to contact you to verify or clarify information. It is helpful to have the patient's medical record in front of you when telephoning a pharmacy with a prescription so that you will have access to information such as allergies, date of birth, and weight. It is also important to document in the record the time and date that

the prescription was phoned in and the name of the person you spoke with at the pharmacy, and it is recommended that you verify the location of the pharmacy. It is helpful to spell out the patient's name, especially if you are recording the information rather than speaking with the pharmacist in person. You might also need to spell out the name of the medication. Be sure to indicate quantity to be dispensed; instructions for taking the medication; how many, if any, refills are allowed; and whether generic substitution is permissible.

Common Errors in Prescription Writing

Almost 70% of provider/patient encounters for acute problems result in the writing of one or more prescriptions. Serious errors can occur, both in writing the prescription and in dispensing the medication. Several studies have identified errors commonly made in the process. These studies have shown that as many as a third of all outpatient prescriptions contain errors. Specific errors fall into these general categories:

- Illegibility of any part of the prescription.
- Omissions: leaving off drug name, strength, or quantity to dispense; minor omissions include not putting patient's name, date, directions for use, or prescriber's name.
- Dose or direction error: exceeding recommended dose or substantial departure from recommended dose; not including indication for PRN medications.
- Legal requirements not met: not including Drug Enforcement Agency (DEA) number on a controlled substance prescription, dispensing quantity above that allowed by state regulation, not spelling out the quantity of a controlled substance, including refills when not allowed by law.
- Unclear quantity prescribed: quantity does not match directions, specifying non-trade-size topical preparations or liquid antibiotics.
- Incomplete directions: not identifying route, quantity to be taken at each dose, frequency of dosing.
- Leading and trailing zeros: not putting a leading zero before a decimal expression of less than one, including a trailing zero after a decimal. Examples are shown in Figure 12–5

Midwestern University
Primary Care Pediatrics
19555 N. 59th Ave.
Glendale, AZ 85308
Phone: 623-572-3000
Fax: 623-572-3400

James E. Meyer, MD
DEA # _____

Debbie D. Sullivan, PA-C
DEA # _____

Name: *Jack Smith* _____   Age: *60* _____

Address: *8104 Palomino Dr.* _____   Date: *xx/xx/xx* _____

Lanoxin `0.125` *mg tabs* `(NOT .125 mg)`
Disp. 30
Sig: ÷ po q am to regulate heart rate

Refill _2_ times   Childproof Container: ☐ yes ☑ no

D Sullivan PAC
_____   _____
Dispense as written   Substitution Permitted

Figure 12–5. (A) Leading zero.

Midwestern University
Primary Care Pediatrics
19555 N. 59th Ave.
Glendale, AZ 85308
Phone: 623-572-3000
Fax: 623-572-3400

James E. Meyer, MD
DEA # _____

Debbie D. Sullivan, PA-C
DEA # _____

Name: *Janet Smith*_____   Age: __*33*_____

Address: *14222 McDonald St.*_____   Date: __*xx/xx/xx*_____

Humulin 70/30
Disp. 10 ml vial
Sig: `13 units` *SQ in am* `(NOT 13.0 units)`

Refill __1__ times   Childproof Container: ☐ yes   ☑ no

_____   *D Sullivan PAC*_____
Dispense as written   Substitution Permitted

Figure 12–5. (B) Trailing zero.

Application Exercise 12.1

The prescriptions that appear in Figures 12–6, 12–7, and 12–8 have errors. Determine what is incorrect, and rewrite the prescription correctly in the blank prescriptions provided.

APPLICATION EXERCISE 12.1 ANSWER

See the correct prescriptions with the corrected information highlighted in Figures 12–9, 12–10, and 12–11.

■ Protecting Your DEA Number

The DEA is the federal agency that regulates controlled substances. To prescribe controlled substances, a provider must register with the DEA and have a unique DEA number. A controlled substance cannot be filled without the provider's DEA number. Because people addicted to controlled substances often forge prescriptions, carefully guard your DEA number to prevent it being used in an unauthorized way. Basic steps to protect your DEA number include the following (text continues on page 168):

Midwestern University
Primary Care Pediatrics
19555 N. 59th Ave.
Glendale, AZ 85308
Phone: 623-572-3000
Fax: 623-572-3400

James E. Meyer, MD   Debbie D. Sullivan, PA-C
DEA # _____   DEA # _____

Name: *Joe Brown* _____   Age: *45* _____
Address: *2626 Michigan ave.* _____   Date: *xx/xx/xx* _____

Accupril
Disp: 30
Sig: ÷ tab po daily for hypertension

Refill _5_ times   Childproof Container: ☑ yes   ☐ no

_____   *D Sullivan PAC* _____
Dispense as written   Substitution Permitted

Figure 12–6. (A) Prescription containing an error.

Midwestern University
Primary Care Pediatrics
19555 N. 59th Ave.
Glendale, AZ 85308
Phone: 623-572-3000
Fax: 623-572-3400

James E. Meyer, MD   Debbie D. Sullivan, PA-C
DEA # _____   DEA # _____

Name: _____   Age: _____
Address: _____   Date: _____

Refill _____ times   Childproof Container: ☐ yes   ☐ no

_____   _____
Dispense as written   Substitution Permitted

Figure 12–6. (B) Identify what is incorrect and write correctly.

Midwestern University
Primary Care Pediatrics
19555 N. 59th Ave.
Glendale, AZ 85308
Phone: 623-572-3000
Fax: 623-572-3400

James E. Meyer, MD   Debbie D. Sullivan, PA-C
    DEA # _____   DEA # _____

Name: *Jacqueline Brown*   Age: _7_
Address: *1007 W. Manzanita*   Date: *xx/xx/xx*

Ritalin LA 20mg tabs
Disp: 30
Sig: ÷ po

Refill __2__ times   Childproof Container: ☑ yes   ☐ no

_____   *DSullivan, PAC*
    Dispense as written   Substitution Permitted

Figure 12–7. (A) Prescription containing errors.

Midwestern University
Primary Care Pediatrics
19555 N. 59th Ave.
Glendale, AZ 85308
Phone: 623-572-3000
Fax: 623-572-3400

James E. Meyer, MD   Debbie D. Sullivan, PA-C
    DEA # _____   DEA # _____

Name: _____   Age: _____
Address: _____   Date: _____

Refill _____ times   Childproof Container: ☐ yes   ☐ no

_____   _____
    Dispense as written   Substitution Permitted

Figure 12–7. (B) Write correctly.

Midwestern University
Primary Care Pediatrics
19555 N. 59th Ave.
Glendale, AZ 85308
Phone: 623-572-3000
Fax: 623-572-3400

James E. Meyer, MD   Debbie D. Sullivan, PA-C

DEA # _____   DEA # _____

Name: *Jason Brown*   Age: *32*
Address: *3701 E. Manor st.*   Date: *xx/xx/xx*

Biaxin
Disp: 30
Sig: ÷ tab BID × 10 days

Refill _Ø_ times   Childproof Container: ☒ yes   ☐ no

_____   *DSullivan PAC*
                                                         _____
Dispense as written   Substitution Permitted

Figure 12–8. (A) A number of items are incorrect.

Midwestern University
Primary Care Pediatrics
19555 N. 59th Ave.
Glendale, AZ 85308
Phone: 623-572-3000
Fax: 623-572-3400

James E. Meyer, MD   Debbie D. Sullivan, PA-C

DEA # _____   DEA # _____

Name: _____   Age: _____
Address: _____   Date: _____

Refill _____ times   Childproof Container: ☐ yes   ☐ no

_____   _____
Dispense as written   Substitution Permitted

Figure 12–8. (B) Write correctly.

Midwestern University
Primary Care Pediatrics
19555 N. 59th Ave.
Glendale, AZ 85308
Phone: 623-572-3000
Fax: 623-572-3400

James E. Meyer, MD
DEA # _____

Debbie D. Sullivan, PA-C
DEA # _____

Name: *Joe Brown* _____   Age: *45* _____

Address: *2626 Michigan ave.* _____   Date: *xx/xx/xx* _____

Accupril `20 mg tabs`
Disp: 30
Sig: ÷ tab po daily for hypertension

Refill __*5*__ times   Childproof Container: ☑ yes   ☐ no

_____   *DSullivan PAC*
                                            _____
Dispense as written   Substitution Permitted

Figure 12–9. Correct prescription for Figure 12–6. The correction is highlighted.

Midwestern University
Primary Care Pediatrics
19555 N. 59th Ave.
Glendale, AZ 85308
Phone: 623-572-3000
Fax: 623-572-3400

James E. Meyer, MD
DEA # _____

Debbie D. Sullivan, PA-C
DEA # ___*DS12345XX*___

Name: *Jacqueline Brown* _____   Age: *7* _____

Address: *1007 W. Manzanita* _____   Date: *xx/xx/xx* _____

Ritalin LA 20 mg tabs
Disp: 30
Sig: ÷ tab po q Am for ADHD. Swallow whole.

Refill __∅__ times   Childproof Container: ☒ yes   ☐ no

_____   *DSullivan PAC*
Dispense as written   Substitution Permitted

Figure 12–10. Correct prescription for Figure 12–7. The corrections are highlighted.

Midwestern University
Primary Care Pediatrics
19555 N. 59th Ave.
Glendale, AZ 85308
Phone: 623-572-3000
Fax: 623-572-3400

James E. Meyer, MD
DEA # _____

Debbie D. Sullivan, PA-C
DEA # _____

Name: *Jason Brown* _____   Age: *32* _____

Address: *3701 E. Manor st.* _____   Date: *xx/xx/xx* _____

Biaxin *500 mg tabs*
Disp: 20 tabs
Sig: ÷ *tab* *po* *BID* × *10 days* *for sinusitis*

Refill ___Ø___ times   Childproof Container: ☒ yes   ☐ no

_____   *DSullivan PAC*
_____

Dispense as written   Substitution Permitted

Figure 12–11. Correct prescription for Figure 12–8. The corrections are highlighted.

- Do not include your DEA number on preprinted prescription pads. Instead, leave a blank line, and write it in only when required for a controlled substance.

- Do not leave prescription pads in examination rooms or in other easily accessible or high-traffic areas. Keep one pad in your pocket, and lock up the rest in a safe and secure place.

- Keep an inventory of the number of prescription pads you have on hand, making it easier to identify whether pads are missing.

- Do not use your DEA number as an identifier. Some pharmacies, suppliers of durable medical equipment, and insurance companies ask for the DEA number as a provider identifier. Some journals use it to obtain access to on-line articles. Using your DEA number for identification increases the risk of misuse and the possibility of forged prescriptions.

- Do not display your DEA certificate. File it in a locked cabinet.

- Limit the number of people who have access to your DEA number. You may allow one trusted nurse or medical assistant access to your DEA number, but it is rarely necessary for everyone in the office to know that number. Instruct office staff to refer all requests for your DEA number directly to you.

Chapter Summary

- Always include the required elements, whether writing a prescription or transmitting by telephone.

- Know and follow state laws and regulations when writing prescriptions for controlled substances.
- Write legibly!
- Avoid dangerous abbreviations.
- Provide an indication for the medication as a safety measure.
- Protect your DEA number against fraudulent use.
- Remember, if it is not documented, it was not done!

Abbreviations

A

A&O	alert & oriented
AB, ab	abortion
Ab	antibody
ABG	arterial blood gas
ac	before meals (ante cibum)
ACTH	adrenocorticotropic hormone
ADA	American Diabetes Association
AD CAVA DIMPLS	Admit, diagnosis, conditions, activity, vital signs, allergies, diet, intervention, medication procedures, labs, special instructions
ADH	antidiuretic hormone (vasopressin)
ad lib	as desired
AFP	alpha-fetoprotein
Ag	antigen
AIDS	acquired immunodeficiency syndrome
AKA	above-knee amputation
alk phos	alkaline phosphatase
ALL	acute lymphocytic leukemia
ALS	amyotrophic lateral sclerosis
AMA	against medical advice
AMI	acute myocardial infarction
AML	acute myelogenous leukemia
ANA	antinuclear antibody
ANS	autonomic nervous system
AP	anteroposterior
ARF	acute renal failure
AVR	aortic valve replacement

B

baso	basophil
BBB	bundle branch block
BID, bid	twice a day
BKA	below-knee amputation
BM	bowel movement
BMI	body mass index
BMR	basal metabolic rate
BP	blood pressure
BPH	benign prostatic hyperplasia
BR	bed rest
BRP	bathroom privileges
BUN	blood urea nitrogen
Bx	biopsy

C

C1, C2, etc.	first cervical vertebra, second cervical vertebra, etc.
C&S	culture and sensitivity
Ca++	calcium
CA	cancer
CAD	coronary artery disease
CAGE	cut down, annoyed, guilty, eye opener
cath	catheterization, catheter
CBC	complete blood count
CC	chief complaint
cc	cubic centimeter
CCU	coronary care unit
CDC	Centers for Disease Control and Prevention
CEA	carcinoembryonic antigen
CHD	coronary heart disease
CHF	congestive heart failure
CK	creatine kinase
C1	chlorine
CLL	chronic lymphocytic leukemia
cm	centimeter
CML	chronic myelogenous leukemia
CMMS	Centers for Medicare and Medicaid Services
CMP	comprehensive metabolic panel
CN	cranial nerve
CNS	central nervous system
c/o	complains of
CO₂	carbon dioxide
COPD	chronic obstructive pulmonary disease
CP	cerebral palsy
CPD	cephalopelvic disproportion
CPK	creatine phosphokinase
CPR	cardiopulmonary resuscitation
CS, C-section	cesarean section
CSF	cerebrospinal fluid
CTA	clear to auscultation
CTS	carpal tunnel syndrome
CT scan, CAT scan	computed tomography scan, computed axial tomography scan
CV	cardiovascular
CVA	cerebrovascular accident

CVD	cerebrovascular disease
CVS	chorionic villus sampling
CXR	chest x-ray film, chest radiograph
cysto	cystoscopy

_D_

d	day or daily
/d	per day
D₅NS	5% dextrose in normal saline (IV solutions)
D&C	dilation and curettage
D&E	dilation and evacuation
DAW	dispense as written
D/C, dc	discharge or discontinue
DDST-II	Denver Developmental Screening Test, 2nd edition
DDX	differential diagnosis
DEA	Drug Enforcement Agency
diff	differential count (white blood cells)
DJD	degenerative joint disease
dL	deciliter
DM	diabetes mellitus
DO	Doctor of Osteopathy
DOA	dead on arrival
DOB	date of birth
DOE	dyspnea on exertion
DPT	diphtheria, pertussis, tetanus
DRE	digital rectal examination
DRG	diagnosis-related group
DTP	diphtheria, tetanus, pertussis
DTR	deep tendon reflexes
DUB	dysfunctional uterine bleeding
DVT	deep vein thrombosis
Dx	diagnosis

_E_

EBL	estimated blood loss
EBV	Epstein-Barr virus
ECF	extracellular fluid
ECG, EKG	electrocardiogram
ECHO	echocardiogram
ED	emergency department
EDC	estimated date of confinement
EEG	electroencephalogram, electroencephalograph
EENT	eyes, ears, nose, and throat
EMG	electromyogram
ENT	ears, nose, and throat
EOM	extraocular movement
eos, eosin	eosinophil
EPSDT	early periodic screening detection and treatment
ERCP	endoscopic retrograde cholangiopancreatography
ERT	estrogen replacement therapy
ESR (SR, sed rate)	erythrocyte sedimentation rate (sedimentation rate)
ESWL	extracorporeal shock-wave lithotripsy

_F_

F	Fahrenheit
FBS	fasting blood sugar
FDA	Food and Drug Administration
FEF	forced expiratory flow
FEV	forced expiratory volume
FH	family history
FHR	fetal heart rate
FHT	fetal heart tone
FOBT	fecal occult blood test
FS	frozen section
FSH	follicle-stimulating hormone
F/U	follow-up
FUO	fever of undetermined origin
FVC	forced vital capacity
Fx	fracture

_G_

g	gram
GB	gallbladder
GC	gonorrhea
GERD	gastroesophageal reflux disease
GH	growth hormone
GI	gastrointestinal
gr	grain
gtt	drops (guttae)
GTT	glucose tolerance test
GU	genitourinary
GYN	gynecology

_H_

H&H	hemoglobin & hematocrit
H&P	history and physical
h, hr	hour
HAV	hepatitis A virus
HBV	hepatitis B virus
HCG	human chorionic gonadotropin
HCl	hydrochloric acid
HCO₃	bicarbonate
HCT, Hct	hematocrit
HDL	high-density lipoprotein
HEENT	head, eyes, ears, nose, and throat
Hg	mercury
HGB, Hgb, Hb	hemoglobin
HgbA₁C	glycosylated hemoglobin A₁
Hib	_Haemophilus influenzae_ type b
HIV	human immunodeficiency virus
HNP	herniated nucleus pulposus (herniated disk)
HPI	history of present illness
HR	heart rate
hs	at bedtime
HSM	hepatosplenomegaly
HSV	herpes simplex virus
Ht	height
HTN	hypertension
HX, Hx	history

_I_

I&D	incision and drainage
I&O	intake and output
IBS	irritable bowel syndrome

ICD-10	International Classification of Diseases-10th Revision		MI	myocardial infarction; mitral insufficiency
ICF	intracellular fluid		mL	milliliter (0.001 liter)
ICP	intracranial pressure		mm	millimeter (0.001 meter; 0.039 inch)
ICS	incentive spirometer		MMR	measles, mumps, rubella
ICU	intensive care unit		mono	monocyte; mononucleosis
ID	intradermal; infectious disease		MRI	magnetic resonance imaging
I&D	incision and drainage		MS	multiple sclerosis; musculoskeletal
Ig	immunoglobulin		MVP	mitral valve prolapse
IM	intramuscular			
inj	injection		_N_	
INR	International Normalized Ratio		Na$^+$	sodium (an electrolyte)
IOP	intraocular pressure		NAD	no acute distress
IPPB	intermittent positive-pressure breathing		NCEP	National Cholesterol Education Program
ITP	idiopathic thrombocytopenia purpura		NIDDM	non–insulin-dependent diabetes mellitus
IUD	intrauterine device		NKDA	no known drug allergies
IUGR	intrauterine growth rate; intrauterine growth retardation		NPH	neutral protamine Hagedorn (insulin)
IV	intravenous		NPO, npo	nothing by mouth (nulla per os)
IVP	intravenous pyelogram		NSAID	nonsteroidal anti-inflammatory drug
_J_			NSVD	normal spontaneous vaginal delivery
JCAHO	Joint Commission on Accreditation of Healthcare Organizations		NVS	neurovascular status
JVD	jugular venous distention		_O_	
			O$_2$	oxygen
_K_			OA	osteoarthritis
K$^+$	potassium (an electrolyte)		OB	obstetrics
kg	kilogram		OB-GYN	obstetrics and gynecology
KUB	kidney, ureter, and bladder		OCP	oral contraceptive pill
			OD	right eye (oculus dexter); overdose
_L_			OOB	out of bed
L	liter		OR	operating room
L1, L2, etc.	first lumbar vertebra, second lumbar vertebra, etc.		ORTH, ortho	orthopedics
LAT, lat	lateral		OS	left eye (oculus sinister)
LDL	low-density lipoprotein		os	mouth; opening; bone
LE	lupus erythematosus; lower extremity		OTC	over the counter
LH	luteinizing hormone		OU	both eyes (oculi unitas)
LLL	left lower lobe		OV	office visit
LLQ	left lower quadrant		oz	ounce
LMP	last menstrual period			
LP	lumbar puncture		_P_	
LPN	licensed practical nurse		P	pulse
L, lt	left		PA	posteroanterior; Physician Assistant
LUQ	left upper quadrant		PAC	premature arterial contraction
lymph	lymphocyte		PA-C	Physician Assistant, Certified
			PAP	Papanicolaou
_M_			PAT	paroxysmal atrial tachycardia
MCH	mean corpuscular hemoglobin		pc	after meals
MCHC	mean corpuscular hemoglobin concentration		PCA	patient-controlled analgesia
MCV	mean corpuscular volume		PCP	_Pneumocystis carinii_ pneumonia
MD	Medical Doctor		PCV	packed cell volume (hematocrit)
met	metastasis		PDR	_Physician's Desk Reference_
mg	milligram (0.001 gram)		PE	physical examination; pulmonary embolus
MG	myasthenia gravis			

PFT	pulmonary function test	SA	sinoatrial (node)
pH	hydrogen ion concentration; level of acidity	SAH	subarachnoid hemorrhage
		SC, sc	subcutaneous
PID	pelvic inflammatory disease	seg	polymorphonuclear neutrophil
PKU	phenylketonuria	SGOT, SGPT	liver function enzyme tests
PMH	past medical history	SIDS	sudden infant death syndrome
PMI	point of maximal intensity, point of maximum impact	sig	signa, instructions for patients
		SLE	systemic lupus erythematosus
PMN, poly	polymorphonuclear neutrophil	SOB	shortness of breath
PMS	premenstrual syndrome	Sp. gr., SG	specific gravity
PND	paroxysmal nocturnal dyspnea	S/P	status post (after)
PNS	peripheral nervous system	SR	sedimentation rate
PO, po	orally, by mouth	staph	staphylococcus
POD	postoperative day	stat	immediately
pp	postprandial (after meals)	STD	sexually transmitted disease
PPD	packs per day	strep	streptococcus
PRN	as required	subcu, subq	subcutaneous
PSA	prostate-specific antigen	SVD	spontaneous vaginal delivery
PT, pro time	prothrombin time	SVN	single volume nubulizer
pt	patient	Sx	signs, symptoms
PT	physical therapy		
PTCA	percutaneous transluminal coronary angiography	*T*	
		T	temperature
PTH	parathyroid hormone	T1, T2, etc.	first thoracic vertebra, second thoracic vertebra, etc.
PTT	partial thromboplastin time		
PUD	peptic ulcer disease	T3	triiodothyronine
PVC	premature ventricular contraction	T4	thyroxine
		T&A	tonsillectomy and adenoidectomy
PVD	peripheral vascular disease		
		TAH	total abdominal hysterectomy
Q		TB	tuberculosis
q	every	Td	tetanus, diphtheria
q2h	every 2 hours	THR	total hip replacement
qam,	every morning	TIA	transient ischemic attack
qd	every day (quaque die)	TID, tid	three times a day
qh	every hour	TKR	total knee replacement
QID, qid	four times a day	TMJ	temporomandibular joint
		TMP/SMX	trimethoprim/sulfamethoxazole
R			
R	respiration	TM	tympanic membrane
RA	rheumatoid arthritis	TNM	tumor, nodes, metastasis
RBC	red blood cell	TPA	tissue plasminogen activator
RDS	respiratory distress syndrome	TPN	total parenteral nutrition
REM	rapid eye movement	TPR	temperature, pulse, and respiration
RF	rheumatoid factor		
RLL	right lower lobe	TSH	thyroid-stimulating hormone
RLQ	right lower quadrant	TUR	transperineal urethral resection
RML	right middle lobe		
RN	registered nurse	TURP	transurethral resection of prostate
R/O	rule out		
ROM	range of motion		
ROS	review of systems	*U*	
RRR	regular rate and rhythm	U	unit
R, rt	right	UA	urinalysis
RTC	return to clinic	UGI	upper gastrointestinal
RUL	right upper lobe	URI	upper respiratory infection
RUQ	right upper quadrant	UTI	urinary tract infection
Rx	prescription, treatment, therapy	UV	ultraviolet
S		*V*	
s̄	without	VCU, VCUG	voiding cystourethrogram
S1, S2, etc.	first sacral vertebra, second sacral vertebra, etc.	VDRL	Venereal Disease Research Laboratory

VLDL	very low-density lipoprotein	**WNL**	within normal limits
VS	vital signs	**Wt**	weight
VSD	ventricular septal defect	**WWE**	well woman examination
VT	ventricular tachycardia		
		_X_	
_W_		x	multiplied by
WBC	white blood cell	**XX**	female sex chromosome
WDWN	well developed, well nourished	**XY**	male sex chromosome

Worksheet Answer Key

Worksheet 1.1 Answers

Part A

A patient presents with a chief complaint of back pain. Below are several statements from the HPI for a chief complaint of back pain. Number them in the order they should appear in the subjective paragraph.

__4___ Pertinent negative associated symptom: The patient denies any trauma.

__5___ Aggravating factor: The pain is worse after standing or walking for more than 20 minutes.

__1___ Onset: The pain started 3 days ago after moving some heavy furniture.

__3___ Pertinent positive associated symptom: The patient has had a tingling sensation in the right buttock area.

__2___ Severity: The pain is described as a dull ache and is rated as a 4/10.

Part B

After the HPI, the past medical history (PMH) should be documented. Place a check beside all statements that are part of the PMH.

_____ There is no family history of heart disease.

_____ The patient smokes 1 pack per day.

__x___ The patient is allergic to penicillin.

_____ The patient works as a mechanic.

__x___ No chronic medical conditions.

__x__ The patient takes Zantac daily.

Part C

Which of the following would be documented as subjective information?
 Circle all that apply.   (**Bold** indicates which ones should be circled.)

vital signs	**family history**	**onset of chief complaint**
history obtained from spouse	complete blood count (CBC) results	
medications	physical exam findings	
information from previous medical records		**review of systems**
x-ray report		

Worksheet 1.2 Answers

These abbreviations were introduced in this chapter. Following each abbreviation, write out the meaning.

S	subjective
O	objective
A	assessment
P	plan
CC	chief complaint
HPI	history of present illness
PMH	past medical history
ROS	review of systems
CBC	complete blood count

Worksheet 2.1 Answers

Part A

Number the following sentences in the order they should appear in the subjective paragraph.

___2_ Onset: The symptoms started 3 days ago.

___3_ Pertinent positive associated symptoms: The patient has had cough and low-grade fever.

___5_ Aggravating/alleviating factors: Over-the-counter cough medication has not decreased his cough.

___1_ Chief complaint: The patient complains of cold symptoms.

___4_ Pertinent negative associated symptoms: The patient has not had increased sputum production or shortness of breath.

Part B

Number the following sentences in the order they should appear in the objective paragraph, according to the usual head-to-toe order.

_5___ The abdomen is soft and nondistended.

_2___ The oropharynx shows some erythema of the posterior pharyngeal wall but no exudates.

_4___ Auscultation of the lungs does not reveal any adventitious breath sounds.

_3___ The neck is supple with full range of motion, and there are no signs of meningeal irritation.

___1__ The skin is warm to touch and without cyanosis.

Worksheet 2.2 Answers

Read the following sentences and determine whether the information is subjective or objective. Place an S (subjective) or an O (objective) in the space provided.

1. S
2. O
3. S
4. O
5. O
6. O
7. S
8. O
9. O
10. S
11. S
12. O
13. O
14. S
15. O
16. O
17. S
18. S
19. O
20. S

Worksheet 2.3 Answers

These abbreviations were introduced in Chapter 2. Beside each, write its meaning.

ECG, EKG	electrocardiogram
BP	blood pressure
HEENT	head, eyes, ears, nose, throat
WBC	white blood count
WNL	within normal limits
CMP	comprehensive metabolic panel
CT	computed tomography
VS	vital signs
Hct	hematocrit
Hgb	hemoglobin

Worksheet 3.1 Answers

1. What is your assessment of the patient in the example?

    One presumptive diagnosis would be tonsillitis.

2. What else would you include in your differential diagnosis?

    Upper respiratory infection (URI), Group A strep, tonsillitis/pharyngitis, and influenza are the most likely diagnoses. Other diagnoses could include mononucleosis and diphtheria.

3. What tests, if any, would you order?

    A rapid strep assay is available in some offices. A throat culture may be sent to the lab. Other tests could include CBC, mono test, throat culture for diphtheria.

Worksheet 3.2 Answers

Fill in the blank using correct medical terminology for the lay terms on the left.

1.	miscarriage	abortion, spontaneous
2.	mole	neoplasm, skin; nevus
3.	nearsightedness	myopia
4.	stiff neck	torticollis
5.	athlete's foot	tinea pedis
6.	hives	urticaria
7.	measles	rubeola
8.	tingling	paresthesias
9.	loss of appetite	anorexia
10.	fear of crowds	ochlophobia
11.	canker sore	aphthous ulcer
12.	navel	umbilicus

Worksheet 3.3 Answers

These abbreviations were introduced in Chapter 3. Beside each, write its meaning.

UTI	urinary tract infection	GI	gastrointestinal
DDX	differential diagnosis	A&O	alert & oriented
PRN, prn	as required	URI	upper respiratory infection
COPD	chronic obstructive pulmonary disease	CMMS	Centers for Medicare and Medicaid Services
CAD	coronary artery disease	d	day or daily
HX, Hx	history	DM	diabetes mellitus
SOB	shortness of breath	GERD	gastroesophageal reflux disease
DOE	dyspnea on exertion	GU	genitourinary
STD	sexually transmitted disease	Ht	height
ROM	range of motion	HTN	hypertension
WDWN	well developed, well nourished	mg	milligram
NAD	no acute distress	MI	myocardial infarction
TM	tympanic membrane	MS	musculoskeletal
PMI	point of maximal intensity	P	pulse
CN	cranial nerve	PA	posteroanterior
DTR	deep tendon reflex	PPD	packs per day
NKDA	no known drug allergies	q	every
JVD	jugular venous distention	R	respirations
HR	heart rate	R/O	rule out
HSM	hepatosplenomegaly	T	temperature
CXR	chest x-ray	Wt	weight
ICD-10	International Classification of Diseases-10th Revision		

Worksheet 4.1 Answers

Part A

Which of the following would be documented in the plan? Circle all that apply. (**bolded** words should be documented)

physical exam findings	information from previous medical records	
patient education	CBC results	r/o ankle fracture
lab and x-ray orders	vital signs	**recommended OTC meds**
review of systems	**referrals**	**follow-up instructions**

Number the following sentences in the suggested order they should appear in the plan by using 1 for tests and referrals, 2 for pharmaceuticals, 3 for patient education, and 4 for follow-up instructions.

Part B

__3__   Discussed the DDX with patient

__1__   Bone densitometry

__2__   Ibuprofen 200 mg 1 or 2 every 6 hours PRN pain

__4__   Follow up in 2 weeks

__1__   CT of chest

__1__   Refer to behavioral health clinic for counseling

__4__   Go to the ED PRN vomiting or increased abdominal pain

__3__   Handout on low back exercises given and explained

__1__   ENT consult

__2__   Albuterol inhaler 1 to 2 puffs every 4–6 hours PRN wheezing.

Worksheet 4.2 Answers

These abbreviations were introduced in Chapter 4. Beside each, write its meaning.

PA	physician assistant
ED	emergency department
D/C	discharge or discontinue
RTC	return to clinic
po	per os (by mouth)
ENT	Ear, nose, and throat

Worksheet 5.1 Answers

1. F
2. F
3. F
4. F
5. T
6. F
7. T
8. F
9. T
10. F

Worksheet 5.2 Answers

These abbreviations were introduced in Chapter 5. Beside each, write its meaning.

DTP	diphtheria, tetanus, pertussis
PAP	Papanicolaou's smear
Hib	*Haemophilus influenzae* Type b
MMR	measles, mumps, rubella
OTC	over the counter
TB	tuberculosis
Td	tetanus, diphtheria
HS, hs	at bedtime

Worksheet 6.1 Answers

1. List three general reasons why a patient would schedule a problem-specific office visit.

    (1) Illness, injury; (2) a new symptom or problem; (3) concerns or questions

2. Mrs. Gonzalez, an established patient, presents to your office with a chief complaint of "right elbow swelling × 2 days."

   Which of the following statements do NOT belong in this problem-specific progress note? Circle all that apply. (**Bold** indicates which ones should be circled.)

   Patient hit her elbow on the corner of a coffee table

   Mother alive and well, 74 years old, HTN × 25 years

   Hospitalized age 22 for pneumonia

   Bursitis, right elbow, secondary to trauma

   Patient denies history of IV drug abuse

3. List six components of a problem-specific progress note. Example: chief complaint.

   (1) HPI; (2) PMH, social history, and family history that are pertinent to the HPI; (3) ROS with pertinent positives and negatives that pertain to the HPI; (4) a focused exam pertinent to the HPI; (5) Assessment; (6) Plan.

4. Give at least four reasons why a patient would be advised to schedule a follow-up visit.

   To discuss (1) test results; (2) his or her visit with a specialist; (3) his or her response to treatment and whether a different course of treatment is needed; (4) a visit to the emergency room or urgent care clinic, (5) hospitalizations and surgeries.

5. Explain the purpose of flow sheets.

   Flow sheets are an excellent "at a glance" method of reviewing the status of a patient's medical condition.

6. Name three conditions for which flow sheets might be a useful tool.

   anticoagulant therapy, diabetes mellitus, hypertension, hyperlipidemia

7. Evaluate the following statements. Place a T for true or an F for false in the space provided.

   _T_ The frequency of periodic monitoring visits depends on the stability of the patient's condition.

   _F_ Use of a checklist to document progress notes is considered fraudulent.

   _F_ A referral is used if you want a second opinion from another health care provider.

   _T_ The referring provider is responsible for transmitting pertinent information to the consulting provider.

   _T_ When patients undergo a minor procedure, they must sign a consent form.

Worksheet 6.2 Answers

These abbreviations were introduced in Chapter 6. Beside each, write its meaning.

CTA	clear to auscultation
RRR	regular rate and rhythm
IV	intravenous
NVS	neurovascular status
TSH	thyroid-stimulating hormone
F/U	follow up
qd	every day
CVA	cerebrovascular accident (stroke)
LDL	low-density lipoprotein
HDL	high-density lipoprotein
I&D	incision and drainage

Worksheet 7.1 Answers

1. List five components of pediatric health maintenance visits.

   (1) growth and developmental screening; (2) laboratory screenings; (3) assess immunization status and immunize as recommended; (4) anticipatory guidance; (5) risk-factor identification

2. List three growth parameters that should be measured and documented from birth to 24 months of age.

   (1) length (or height); (2) weight; (3) head circumference

3. Sexually active pediatric patients should be screened for which of the following? Circle the correct answers. (**Bold** indicates which ones should be circled.)

anemia	galactosemia	**urinalysis**
lead	**STDs**	

4. Name three widely used resources available from the CDC.

   (1) growth charts; (2) BMI charts; (3) recommended immunization schedules

5. Which statement is TRUE? Statement B.

   a) The pediatric physical examination may be

completed in any order and documented in any order.

b) The pediatric physical examination may be performed in order and should be documented in head-to-toe order.

Worksheet 7.2 Answers

These abbreviations were introduced in Chapter 7. Beside each, write its meaning.

EPSDT	early periodic screening detection and treatment
BMI	body mass index
CDC	Centers for Disease Control and Prevention
DDST-II	Denver Developmental Screening Test, 2nd edition
PKU	phenylketonuria

Worksheet 8.1 Answers

1. List the components of the adult health maintenance examination.

    Risk-factor identification

    Laboratory and diagnostic screening tests

    Immunization status

    Patient education and counseling

2. List five of the risk factors that should be asked about in the personal history.

    Any five of these: exercise, diet, alcohol, tobacco use, other substance abuse, sexual history, blood transfusions, safety, domestic violence, dental, psychiatric, occupational history

3. What are the four questions that make up the CAGE questionnaire?

    Have you ever felt the need to cut down on drinking?

    Have people annoyed you by criticizing your drinking?

    Have you ever felt guilty about your drinking?

    Have you ever taken a drink first thing in the morning to steady your nerves or get rid of a hangover?

4. You are seeing a 68-year-old woman for her annual WWE. The patient has a history of hypertension and a family history of glaucoma. Based on general screening recommendations, personal risk factors, age, and gender, list at least five screening exams that could be ordered for this patient.

    Any of the following: total cholesterol, flexible sigmoidoscopy, colonoscopy, digital rectal exam, FOBT, EKG, CMP, VDRL, glaucoma screening, pelvic exam, PAP, breast exam, mammogram, bone density screening.

5. You are seeing a 52-year-old man for his annual health maintenance visit. List two specific physical examination components and at least three screening tests that could be ordered for this patient.

    Any of these: prostate exam, check for inguinal hernia, rectal exam, digital rectal exam, FOBT, flexible sigmoidoscopy, EKG, total cholesterol, VDRL.

Worksheet 8.2 Answers

These abbreviations were introduced in Chapter 8. Beside each, write its meaning.

CAGE	cut down, annoyed, guilty, eye opener
HIV	human immunodeficiency virus
WWE	well woman exam
ANA	antinuclear antibody
FBS	fasting blood sugar
FOBT	fecal occult blood test
HgbA$_{1C}$	glycosylated hemoglobin A$_1$
RF	rheumatoid factor
VDRL	Venereal Disease Research Laboratory

Worksheet 9.1 Answers

1. Using the example below, identify the elements of an admit note.

    Admit note: Mr. Caruso is a 52-year-old Hispanic man **(identifying data)** who developed chest pain, difficulty breathing, and nausea 4 hours ago **(reason for admission).** His past medical history is significant for hypertension **(pertinent medical history).** He takes Vasotec 10 mg daily. He is not allergic to any medications **(medications and allergies).** On physical examination, he is alert and oriented and appears anxious. He is pale but not cyanotic. Vital signs are BP 138/98, P 110, R 20. HEENT is unremarkable. Neck supple, no JVD. No adventitious breath sounds. Heart is tachycardic but regular with a rate of 110 **(pertinent physical exam findings).** Chest x-ray does not reveal any consolidation or effusion. EKG shows acute ischemic changes consistent with an acute inferior infarct. Troponin I level is elevated at 2.3 **(pertinent laboratory data)**. Impression is acute inferior MI **(admitting diagnosis)**. Mr. Caruso is admitted to the cardiac care unit for IV thrombolytic therapy and supportive care **(summary of treatment plan)**. H&P done and dictated **(H&P done and documented)**.

2. Beside each letter, write the work that represents what should be included in admission orders.

A	admit	D	diet
D	diagnosis	I	interventions
C	condition	M	medication
A	activity	P	procedures
V	vital signs	L	laboratory studies
A	allergies	S	special instructions

3. List three liquids allowed on a clear liquid diet.

   Any of the following: broth, gelatin, tea, apple juice, cranberry juice, grape juice, Pedialyte, Gatorade, clear sodas such as lemon-lime or ginger ale

4. List three liquids or foods allowed on a full liquid diet.

   Any of the following: coffee, milkshake, ice cream, sherbet, soups, oatmeal, cream of wheat, grits, gravy, dark sodas such as colas, orange juice, grapefruit juice, pineapple juice

5. List three foods allowed on a soft diet.

   Any of the following: oatmeal, mashed or baked potatoes, bananas, scrambled eggs, soft bread or rolls, applesauce, gelatin, puddings

Worksheet 9.2 Answers

H&P	history and physical	INR	International Normalized Ratio
JCAHO	Joint Commission on Accreditation of Healthcare Organizations	TNM	tumor, nodes, metastasis
RLL	right lower lobe	OR	operating room
dL	deciliter	S/P	status post (after)
BR	bed rest	I&O	intake and output
BRP	bathroom privileges	ADA	American Diabetes Association

OOB	out of bed	NCEP	National Cholesterol Education Program
NPO	nothing by mouth	PT	prothrombin time; physical therapy
SVN	single-volume nebulizer	PTT	partial thromboplastin time
D₅NS	5% dextrose in normal saline (IV solution)		
H&H	hemoglobin and hematocrit		
AP	anteroposterior		
CEA	carcinoembryonic antigen		
TID, tid	three times daily		
ICS	incentive spirometer		
IM	intramuscular		
PCA	patient-controlled analgesia		

AD CAVA DIMPLS admit, diagnosis, condition, activity, vital signs, allergies, diet, interventions, medications, procedures, labs, special instructions

Worksheet 10.1 Answers

1. List several questions that should be answered daily for postoperative patients.

   Any of the following: Is the patient getting adequate pain relief? Has bowel function returned? Can the activity level be advanced? Can the diet be advanced? Can any staples, sutures, or drains be removed? Are any laboratory, radiographic, or other diagnostic studies needed? Does the patient have any complaints or new problems? Are there any consultations or special services? Is the patient nearing discharge?

2. A postoperative patient has been on a full liquid diet for the past 24 hours. He now has full bowel sounds and says he is hungry. Write an order for a change in diet.

   Possible answers: soft diet, regular diet as tolerated, advance diet as tolerated

3. List seven components of a procedure note.

   (1) name of procedure; (2) indication for procedure; (3) consent; (4) type of anesthesia; (5) details of procedure; (6) findings; (7) complications.

4. List at least five components of an operative note.

Any of the following: date, name of procedure, indication, surgeon, surgical assistant, anesthesia, preoperative diagnosis, postoperative diagnosis, specimens, estimated blood loss, drains, complications, disposition

5. List at least five components of a delivery note.

Any of the following: type of delivery, estimated gestational age of fetus, viability of fetus, sex, 1 and 5 minute Apgar scores, weight, time of delivery of placenta, lacerations, episiotomies, estimated blood loss, condition of mother after delivery

6. List the four Ws that could be sources of postoperative fever.

wind, wound, water, walk

Worksheet 10.2 Answers

These abbreviations were introduced in Chapter 10. Beside each, write its meaning.

POD	postoperative day
EBL	estimated blood loss
NSVD	normal spontaneous vaginal delivery
DVT	deep vein thrombosis

Worksheet 11.1 Answers

1. List three components of a discharge order.

Any of the following: wound care, lifting and amount allowed, bathing, swimming

2. List three components that should be addressed when instructing a patient on activity at the time of a hospital discharge.

Any of the following: disposition, activity, diet, medications, follow-up instructions

3. List 10 components of a discharge summary.

Any of the following:

date of admission	date of discharge	admitting diagnosis
discharge diagnosis	attending physician	consulting physicians
procedures	pertinent history	results of laboratory studies
pertinent exam findings	hospital course	condition at discharge
disposition	medications	follow-up instructions
problem list		

Worksheet 11.2 Answers

These abbreviations were introduced in Chapter 11. Beside each, write its meaning.

AMA	against medical advice
UA	urinalysis
BM	bowel movement

Worksheet 12.1 Answers

These abbreviations were introduced in Chapter 12. Beside each, write its meaning. Also identify which abbreviations are considered "dangerous" when writing prescriptions.

DEA	Drug Enforcement Agency
TMP/SMX	trimethoprim/sulfamethoxazole
AS	left ear
DAW	dispense as written
ac	before meals
BID, bid	twice daily
U	units
AD	right ear
OD	right eye
OS	left eye
OU	both eyes
HS	half strength
TIW	three times weekly
sig	signa, or instructions for patients
gtt	drops
TID, tid	three times a day
QOD	every other day

Chapter 1

Ballweg R, Stolberg S, Sullivan EM. Physician Assistant, 3rd ed. Philadelphia: W.B. Saunders, 2003.

Bardes CL. Essential Skills in Clinical Medicine. Philadelphia: F.A. Davis, 1996.

Bickley LS, Hoekelman RA. Bate's Guide to Physical Examination and History Taking, 8th ed. Philadelphia: Lippincott, 2003.

Coulehan JL, Block MR. The Medical Interview: Mastering Skills for Clinical Practice. Philadelphia: F.A. Davis, 1997.

Crawford G. Guide to Effective Communication. Physician's Financial News. New York: Rogers US Publishing, 2003.

Gomella LG, Haist SA. Clinician's Pocket Reference, 9th ed. San Francisco: McGraw-Hill, 2002.

Kettenbach G. Writing SOAP Notes, 2nd ed. Philadelphia: F.A. Davis, 1995.

Pagano MP. Communicating Effectively in Medical Records: A Guide for Physicians. Newbury Park, CA: Sage, 1992.

Roach WH. Medical Records and the Law, 3rd ed. Gaithersburg, MD: Aspen Publications, 1998.

Saunders CS. Enhancing your practice: Tips for better history-taking. Patient Care Online. June 2002; 8.

Chapter 2: See Chapter 1.

Chapter 3

Ballweg R, Stolberg S, Sullivan EM. Physician Assistant, 3rd ed. Philadelphia: W.B. Saunders, 2003.

Centers for Medicare and Medicaid Services (CMMS). Diagnosis coding: Using the ICD-9-CM. [on-line]. Available at http//www.cms.hhs Accessed November 2, 2002.

Gomella LG, Haist SA. Clinician's Pocket Reference, 9th ed. San Francisco: McGraw-Hill, 2002.

International Classification of Diseases, 9th Revision, Clinical Modification (ICD-9-CM). Los Angeles: Practice Management Information Corporation, 2002.

Raftery AT, Lim E. Churchill's Pocketbook of Differential Diagnosis. Philadelphia: Harcourt Publishers; 2001.

Smith DS. Field Guide to Bedside Diagnosis. Philadelphia: Lippincott, Williams and Wilkins, 1999.

van Bemmel JH, Musen MA, eds. Handbook of Medical Informatics [on-line]. Available at http//www.mieur.nl/ mihandbook/r_3_2/handbook/homepage_self.htm Accessed November 3, 2002.

Wasson JH. The Common Symptom Guide, 5th ed. San Francisco: McGraw-Hill, 2002.

Chapter 4

Ballweg R, Stolberg S, Sullivan EM. Physician Assistant, 3rd ed. Philadelphia: W.B. Saunders, 2003.

Bickley LS, Hoekelman RA. Bate's Guide to Physical Examination and History Taking, 8th ed. Philadelphia: Lippincott, 2003.

Labus JB, Lauber AA. Patient Education and Preventive Medicine. Philadelphia: W.B. Saunders, 2001.

Roach WH. Medical Records and the Law, 3rd ed. Gaithersburg, MD: Aspen Publications, 1998.

Woolf SH, Jonas S, Lawrence RS, eds. Health Promotion and Disease Prevention in Clinical Practice. Philadelphia: Williams & Wilkins, 1996.

Chapter 5

Bartholomew WG. Informed consent, parental permission, and assent in pediatric practice: A document presented to the American Academy of Pediatrics' Committee on Bioethics in 1985; revisited and reaffirmed in 1995 [on-line]. Available at http//www.cirp.org/library/ethics/ AAP/ Accessed October 23, 2002.

Bickley LS, Hoekelman RA. Bate's Guide to Physical Examination and History Taking, 8th ed. Philadelphia: Lippincott, 2003.

Boren SD. Medicare B bulletin: Improving medical record documentation [on-line]. Available at http:// www.chiro.org/documentation/ABSTRACTS/Improvi ng_Medical_Documentation.PDF Accessed October 15, 2002.

Labus JB, Lauber AA. Patient Education and Preventive Medicine. Philadelphia: WB Saunders, 2001.

Rakel RE. Textbook of Family Practice, 6th ed. Philadelphia: W.B. Saunders, 2002.

Roach WH. Medical Records and the Law, 3rd ed. Gaithersburg, MD: Aspen Publications, 1998.

Savage P. A book that changed my practice: Problem-oriented medical records. BMJ 2001; 322:275 [on-line]. Available at http//www.bmj.com Accessed February 28, 2003.

Chapter 6

Bickley LS, Hoekelman RA. Bate's Guide to Physical Examination and History Taking, 8th ed. Philadelphia: Lippincott, 2003.

Labus JB, Lauber AA. Patient Education and Preventive Medicine. Philadelphia: WB Saunders, 2001.

Rakel RE. Textbook of Family Practice, 6th ed. Philadelphia: W.B. Saunders, 2002.

Roach WH. Medical Records and the Law, 3rd ed. Gaithersburg, MD: Aspen Publications, 1998.

Spraycar, M. Stedman's Medical Dictionary. Baltimore: Williams & Wilkins; 1995.

University of Southern California – Bioethics Discussion Pages. Informed Consent [on-line]. Available at http//www-hsc.usc.edu/~mbernste/ethics. informed_consent.html Accessed January 14, 2003.

Chapter 7

American Academy of Pediatrics website: http://www.aap.org

Behrman RE, Kliegman RM. Nelson's Essentials of Pediatrics, 4th ed. WB Saunders: Philadelphia, 2002.

Bickley LS, Hoekelman RA. Bate's Guide to Physical Examination and History Taking, 8th ed. Philadelphia: Lippincott, 2003.

Centers for Disease Control and Prevention website: http://www.cdc.gov

Labus JB, Lauber AA. Patient Education and Preventive Medicine. Philadelphia: WB Saunders, 2001.

Chapter 8

Bickley LS, Hoekelman RA. Bate's Guide to Physical Examination and History Taking, 8th ed. Philadelphia: Lippincott, 2003.

Centers for Disease Control and Prevention website: http://www.cdc.gov

Labus JB, Lauber AA. Patient Education and Preventive Medicine. Philadelphia: WB Saunders, 2001.

Noble J, et al. Textbook of Primary Care Medicine, 3rd ed. St. Louis: Mosby, 2001.

US Preventive Task Force. Guide to Clinical Preventive Services, 3rd ed. Baltimore: Lippincott, Williams & Wilkins, 2003.

Chapter 9

Bardes CL. Essential Skills in Clinical Medicine. Philadelphia: F.A. Davis, 1996.

Gomella LG, Haist SA. Clinician's Pocket Reference, 9th ed. San Francisco: McGraw-Hill, 2002.

Kettenbach G. Writing SOAP Notes, 2nd ed. Philadelphia: F.A. Davis, 1995.

Pagano MP. Communicating Effectively in Medical Records: A Guide for Physicians. Newbury Park, CA: Sage, 1992.

Roach WH. Medical Records and the Law, 3rd ed. Gaithersburg, MD: Aspen Publications, 1998.

Chapter 10: See Chapter 9.

Chapter 11: See Chapter 9.

Chapter 12

Ballweg R, Stolberg S, Sullivan EM. Physician Assistant, 3rd ed. Philadelphia: W.B. Saunders, 2003.

Bardes CL. Essential Skills in Clinical Medicine. Philadelphia: F.A. Davis, 1996.

Federal Drug Administration website. Available at http://www.fda.gov

Gomella LG, Haist SA. Clinician's Pocket Reference, 9th ed. San Francisco: McGraw-Hill, 2002.

Howell RR, Jones KW. Prescription-writing errors and markers: The value of knowing the diagnosis. Fam Med 25(2); 104-106, 1993.

Institute for Safe Medicine Practices website. Available at http://www.ismp.org

Meyer TA. Improving the quality of the order-writing process for inpatient orders and outpatient prescriptions. Am J Health Syst Pharm 57(S4); S18-S22, 2000.

Morse LJ. Misuse of DEA numbers. New Engl J Med 337(20); 1478-1479, 1997.

National Coordinating Council for Medication Error Reporting and Prevention. Recommendations to reduce medication errors associated with verbal medication orders and prescriptions. Available online at http://www.mccmerp.org/rec_010220.htm

Shaughnessy AF, Nickel RO. Prescription-writing patterns and errors in a family medicine residency program. J Fam Pract 29(3); 290-295, 1989.

Teichman PG, Caffee AE. Prescription Writing to Maximize Patient Safety. Fam Pract Manage, July/August 2002. Available at www.aafp.org/fpm

Winslow EH, et al.. Legibility and completeness of physicians' handwritten medication orders. Heart Lung 26(2); 158-164, 1997.

Index

Note: Page numbers followed by the letter b refer to boxed material; those followed by f refer to figures; those followed by t refer to tables.

Subjective Information

Chief complaint: Main reason the patient is seeking care.

HPI: 7 cardinal attributes of CC (onset, location, character, severity, associated signs and symptoms, aggravating factors, alleviating factors).

PMH: Current and/or chronic medical conditions, surgeries, current medications, allergies, immunization status, health maintenance status, preventive care; for females—obstetric and gynecologic history.

FH: Age and current health condition of living parents, siblings, and children; for family members who are deceased—age at death and cause; presence of diseases with a familial tendency.

SH: Marital status, occupation, or student status; living arrangements; education; sexual orientation; habits such as tobacco, alcohol, or drug use.

Psychiatric history: Current mental state, history of depression or other mental disorders, history of suicide threat or attempt.

Cultural history: Belief system as to cause of illness; family dynamics and authority within family; spiritual/religious practices; taboos.

Review of systems—See back of card.

Discharge Orders

- Disposition
- Activity level
- Diet
- Medications
- Follow-up instructions

S: (Subjective): Patient's history. Includes CC, HPI, PMH, family history, social history, other pertinent history, and ROS.

O: (Objective): Physical examination findings, results of diagnostic studies. Examination is documented in the following order: general information, vital signs, skin, HEENT, neck, chest (includes lungs), cardiovascular, abdomen, genitourinary, musculoskeletal, and neurological.

A: Assessment, or the diagnosis. Includes the primary diagnosis and any secondary diagnoses that impact the patient's current state.

P: Plan of care. Includes pharmacological treatment, nonpharmacological interventions, follow-up care, referrals, diagnostic testing, and patient education.

Admission Orders

A — Admit to
D — Diagnosis
C — Condition
A — Activity level
V — Vital sign frequency
A — Allergies
D — Diet order
I — Interventions
M — Medications
P — Procedures
L — Laboratory or diagnostic studies
S — Special instructions

Review of Systems Questions

General: weight gain or loss, activity level, fever, chills, sweats.
Skin: any lesions and size, color, location, characteristics, recent changes.
HEENT: change in hearing, vision, smell, taste; pain or discomfort in ears, eyes, nose, throat, sinuses; persistent or uncharacteristic headaches; nasal discharge, change in voice.
Neck: swollen glands or other areas of swelling; restriction of movement.
Respiratory: shortness of breath; cough; dyspnea on exertion; hemoptysis; orthopnea.
CV: chest pain with or without exertion; chest wall pain; venous distention; swelling of feet and/or hands.
GI: change in appetite; difficulty chewing or swallowing; nausea; vomiting; diarrhea; constipation; cramping; bloating; indigestion; blood in stool; hemorrhoids.
GU: pain with urination, hesitancy; frequency; hematuria.
Reproductive: Female: irregular menses; painful menses; vaginal pain or discharge; dyspareunia; **Male:** penile discharge; testicular or scrotal pain or swelling.
MS: range of motion of joints; joint pain or swelling; redness or warmth of a joint.
Hematological: easy bruising; bleeding from gums; delayed wound healing; recurrent infections.
Psychiatric: affective or personality disorders; depressed mood; sleep disturbances; suicidal ideation; hallucination; illusions; delusions; substance abuse.

Physical Examination

- General Information (patient identifier, such as gender, age, and race)
- Vital signs, height and weight, very brief mental status description
- Skin
- HEENT (head, eyes; ears; nose and throat)
- Neck
- Chest (including lungs)
- Cardiovascular
- Abdomen
- Genitourinary
- Musculoskeletal
- Neurological

Discharge Summary

- Date of admission
- Date of discharge
- Admitting diagnosis
- Discharge diagnosis
- Attending physician
- Referring/consulting physician(s)
- Procedure
- Brief history, examination, and laboratory findings
- Hospital course
- Condition at discharge
- Discharge medications
- Discharge instructions and follow-up
- Problem list

Procedure note: name, indication, consent, anesthesia, details of procedure, findings, complications.

Operative note: date of procedure, name of procedure, indication for procedure, surgeon, surgical assistant(s), anesthesia, preoperative diagnosis, postoperative diagnosis, specimens, EBL, drains, complications, dispositions.

Delivery note: Type of delivery, estimated gestational age of fetus, viability of fetus, gender, Apgar scores at 1 and 5 minutes, weight, delivery of placenta, number of vessels in cord, lacerations or episiotomy, EBL, condition of mother.